I0040480

The Secret Ledger of an
Early Texas Doctor

The Secret Ledger of an Early Texas Doctor

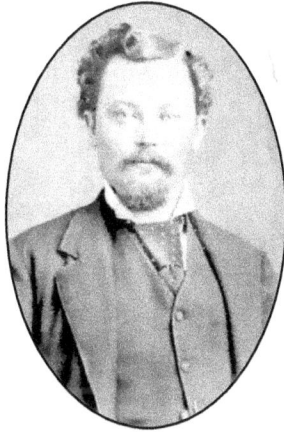

Dr. William Joseph Calhoun Lawrence
and the "Base, Mean, Low-Down, 'Trifeling,'
Lying, Lazy, Hog-Thieving, Indolent, Dogon',
Chisel-Fisted, Cheating, Worthless, Insignificant,
'Contemptable,' Wife-Abusing, Wife-Deserting,
Wife-Neglecting, Diabolical, Cowardly, Dastardly, Loafing,
Sponging, Filthy Scamps, Poltroons, Scoundrels, Puppies,
Rascals, Bad Ones, Dead-Heads, Fools, Bastards,
Reprobates, Sons of Bitches,
'Bouncing Baby Boys Without any Papa'"
And Others of Our Noble Texas Ancestors

By Egon Richard Tausch

With Facsimiles from the Original

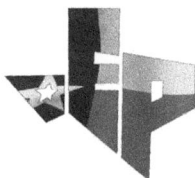

Copyright © 2000
By Phyllis Keil Tausch
Published By Eakin Press
An Imprint of Wild Horse Media Group
P.O. Box 331779
Fort Worth, Texas 76163
1-817-344-7036
www.EakinPress.com
ALL RIGHTS RESERVED
1 2 3 4 5 6 7 8 9
ISBN-10: 1-57168-461-1
ISBN-13: 978-1-57168-461-5

Library of Congress Cataloging-in-Publication Data
Tausch, Egon Richard
   The secret ledger of an early Texas doctor: Dr. William Joseph
Calhoun Lawrence and the base, mean, low-down, trifeling, lying, lazy,
hog-thieving, indolent, dogon', chisel-fisted, cheating, worthless,
insignificant, contemptable, wife-abusing, wife-deserting, wife-neglecting, diabolical, cowardly, dastardly, loafing, sponging, filthy scamps,
poltroons, scoundrels, puppies, rascals, bad ones, dead-heads, fools,
bastards, reprobates, sons of bitches, bouncing baby boys without any
papa / by Egon Richard Tausch.– 1st ed.
      95 p. : ill. ; 23 cm.
   Includes bibliographical references (p. 89-90) and index.
   ISBN 13: 978-1-57168-461-5 (pbk. : alk. paper)
   ISBN 10: 1-57168-461-1 (pbk. : alk. paper)
   1. Lawrence, William Joseph Calhoun, 1850-1884. 2. Physicians--
Texas--Miscellanea. 3. Physicians--Texas--Biography. 4. Medicine--
Texas--History--19th century. I. Title
R154.L335 T38 2000
610/.92 B 21   00062280

To my aunt,
Jane Day Briggs Rambie,
who preserved and gave me
the Ledger kept by her maternal grandfather
(my maternal great-grandfather), that my
inordinate pride of Texian ancestry would be
tempered with reality and wit.

NOTE:
None of the names herein have been changed to
protect the allegedly guilty.

Contents

I.

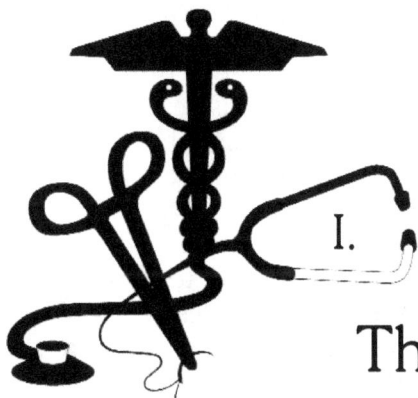

The Setting for a
Texas Son

Leo Tolstoy popularized the debate as to whether history was made by great men and women, or whether these colossi were merely forced on the stage by inevitable Great Events, Shifts, and Movements.

But what about mundane life in the past, and the ordinary men and women who either created or were created by history? For that we have to turn to the writings of mostly unremembered people—diaries, business records, correspondence—most of which lack the scope, eloquence, wisdom, or coherence of Burke's *Reflections on the Revolution in France,* Caesar's *Commentaries,* or Churchill's *History of the English Speaking People.* Statistics (census reports, customs receipts, economic reports, etc.) tend to be as dry as . . . well, statistics. And as misleading.

Rarely do we find a revealing document like *Pepys' Diary* of ordinary life in seventeenth-century London, written by an ordinary man living such a life. And sometimes the more accurate and even-handed the account, the more boring the result. Occasionally we need a diarist of strong opinions, quirky attitudes, malicious wit, and even downright bigotry in order to experience the spicy *flavor* of history.

Which leads to the secret ledger of Dr. William Joseph Calhoun Lawrence, never before published, and unseen by anyone other than his direct descendants for over a hundred years.

1

Dr. Lawrence (born 1850) was a general practitioner in Anderson County, Texas, from the 1870s until his death in a mutually fatal shootout with his cousin over a pair of boys' trousers, on December 2, 1884, at the age of thirty-four.

Dr. Lawrence's father, William Howard Lawrence (March 14, 1808–December 6, 1871), moved to Texas from Aiken, South Carolina, in 1836. Since that up-country town was exclusively an elegant summer-home for rich Charlestonians escaping the fevers raging through the seaport town during that season, it is probably safe to say that Lawrence belonged to that class, and might even have been descended from the Laurence family, prominent French Huguenot settlers of Charleston. His birth is recorded at the Methodist Church in Aiken.

W. H. Lawrence's journey to Texas might have been inspired by Colonel Travis' desperate call from the doomed Alamo. Or perhaps he was just an adventurer—or had other motives for leaving South Carolina quickly.

The first immigrants to Texas from the United States originally settled under Stephen F. Austin, who was granted a charter by the Mexican government of the time, operating under that country's Constitution of 1824. Mexico believed that Texas, an area rich in natural resources, was underpopulated and could not contribute to Mexico's economy. American settlers came by the thousands, many intending to send for their extended families later. The original scattered colonies of Spanish and Mexican inhabitants were, on the whole, happy to see their region grow with immigrants.

Gen. Antonio Lopez de Santa Anna took over the government of Mexico in 1833, and promptly repudiated its constitution. This action would prohibit further immigration, thus dividing families and restricting the civil rights of American, as well as Mexican, Texans. Most of Mexico rose in rebellion against him. He crushed Yucatan and Zacatecas, and marched on the combined state of Tejas y Coahuila. The latter region fell quickly, but Texas continued to oppose Santa Anna, at first as dissident Mexicans. When resistance as such appeared futile, especially after the fall of the Alamo, Texas declared its independence.

William Howard Lawrence fought with the Texas Army before and during the Battle of San Jacinto. The battle was one-sided—Texans suffered thirty-nine casualties, while Santa Anna suffered 1,360 casualties plus his own capture—and Texas independence was secured. Like other soldiers, Lawrence was given a large parcel of land by the grateful new republic.

Republic of Texas document No. 2776, dated April 6, 1838, records "that William Lawrence having served faithfully and honorably for the term of twelve months from the tenth day of May 1836 until the third day of June 1837 and having been honorably discharged from the army is entitled to twelve hundred eighty acres bounty land, for which this is his certificate." Since one year's service was required for a land grant, only the last twelve months were recorded. As did most of the recipients of such "bounties," Lawrence sold his land almost immediately. The reasons for quick sales were numerous: the situation of the land available was not always ideal, many former soldiers had debts to pay, many would have to leave the land to return east to bring their families, some had never intended to stay in Texas in the first place, and a few preferred to live in cities (though there were precious few towns in Texas at the time). Lawrence's intent was to return to South Carolina, marry, begin a family, then settle in Texas permanently. The extreme scarcity of unmarried women in East Texas would have encouraged this plan.

Lawrence's land grant was sold to John Toliver and Joseph Harlan on April 6, 1838—the same date the land was awarded—at Houston, Texas (at the time, a town so small it was not even recorded on most maps of Texas).

After the War for Texas Independence, the elder Lawrence returned to South Carolina and married Clarissa Moody Givens, born March 11, 1818, in Nashville, Tennessee. Lawrence was ten years older than his young bride, which was not uncommon at the time. Lawrence's son, whose ledger is the subject of this book, was thirty when he married; his wife had just turned sixteen. It was expected that the groom be well settled in his trade or profession and prosperous enough to support a family while the bride, usually having no trade and being dependent on her family, was still innocent (and had plenty of time to bear as many children as possible). Also, a grown, unmarried woman—even a widow—was considered a threat to the social fabric, unless she was a very respectable, confirmed "spinster."

Today, the media dwell with pity on teenage mothers ("children having children"), despite the fact that most of our female ancestors married and bore children as teenagers.

William Howard and Clarissa Lawrence eventually had three children: William Joseph Calhoun (born 1850), Musadora Martha (born 1854 and died two years later), and Mary Clementine.

Lawrence returned with his wife to Texas in 1845, while Texas was still a republic and had not yet joined the United States. Lawrence bought 543½ acres of land near Mound Prairie, in what was soon to be named Anderson County. This East Texas county, between the Neches and Trinity rivers, was the center of the prosperous plantation country, with its seat at the town of Palestine, though the nearest city of any substance was Galveston, on the Gulf of Mexico, over 200 miles away. Cotton, livestock, and all the supporting artisans, mechanics, and merchants supplied the basis of the economy. After the war of 1861-1865, the region rapidly declined. Mound Prairie, named after an Indian burial ground, was reduced to a ghost town for many years, though Anderson County itself was later revived by livestock breeding, the bountiful timber, and, of course, the discovery and exploitation of oil. Economics and politics of the area would affect the Lawrence family profoundly.

The political life of Anderson County was homogeneous. Everyone of note was a Democrat, a party which at the time represented conservatism and states' rights. The Whig Party had virtually died out, being based originally on disapproval of former U.S. President Andrew Jackson. The new Republican Party had no followers in Texas. The American Party, called Know-Nothings for their secretive responses, was dedicated to keeping out immigrants—an absurdity in underpopulated Texas. Though that party had some followers in South and Central Texas, where German immigrants predominated, its only accomplishment was to solidify the Texas-Germans as devoted Democrats, like almost everyone else.

Texans of European descent had for years formed an overwhelming majority of the state's voters. Although throughout Texas (as in all the states) only non-black males could vote, their opinions reflected those of their families. Property ownership was no longer a requirement for voting, literacy and poll taxes would not become requirements for over a half-century, and every non-black immigrant in Texas was instantly a citizen of the state and the U.S. with the right to vote. African-American slaves were a small minority, free blacks a tiny minority, and massive immigration from Mexico did not begin until after the turn of the next century. The Spanish and Texas-Mexican population which remained from before the Texas Revolution was mostly amalgamated with the Southern culture, at least in Central and East Texas. Most later Texas Confederate regiments had a significant minority of Hispanic officers and enlisted men, and one of their number, Santos Benavides of Laredo, became a renowned colonel and (provisional) Confederate general.

The two most important contested elections, in Anderson County as elsewhere, occurred in the year of 1860. The first was for the president of the United States, for which there were four candidates. The official Democratic Party nominated Stephen A. Douglas of Illinois. This pending nomination caused the Southern wing of the party to meet in a rump convention in South Carolina, which nominated a committed supporter of states' rights and of the secession of the South, U.S. Vice President (and later Confederate General) James C. Breckinridge of Kentucky. In an effort to reach a compromise between South and North, a new "Constitutional Union" Party was founded, with John Bell, also of Kentucky, as its candidate. The new Republican Party, whose first try for the presidency in 1856, under John C. Fremont of California, was a disaster, now chose Abraham Lincoln of Illinois as its candidate.

In the eyes of most Southerners and Southwesterners, the Republican Party stood for the immediate abolition of black slavery, for strengthening the central government, and for the (unconstitutional) protection of Northern manufacturers through high tariffs, which would greatly harm the agricultural South, relying, as it did, on the importation of finished goods from Europe.

Although Abraham Lincoln denied that he was an abolitionist—he merely wished to prevent the expansion of slavery into previously free states and territories—Texans remembered that as a congressman Lincoln had vociferously opposed Texas as a new state, and later opposed the Mexican War of 1847, which Texans had regarded as the only means to prevent Santa Anna's intermittent incursions into South Texas and the dictator's continued claims that South Texas still belonged to Mexico.

Not having achieved any noticeable support in the South, the Republican Party distributed no ballots for Lincoln in Texas. Similarly, Douglas, the "Northern Democrat," was not on the ballot. Ballots were, at the time, printed and distributed by the parties themselves, rather than governments.

Nevertheless, the election results in Anderson County were indicative of its solidarity. The ardent Secessionist John C. Breckinridge received 853 votes, or 92.4%. Bell, the compromise candidate, won only 113 votes.

Because each of the four candidates received almost equal shares of the votes in the combined states, Abraham Lincoln, who carried the most populous Northern states, became president of the U.S., with the smallest plurality in history. This added to the disaffection of the South in general, and Anderson County, Texas, in particular.

The movement for secession quickly picked up momentum in the state. The Secession Convention soon passed its Ordinance of Secession, led, in part, by Representative Gustav Schleicher, a Hill-Country German. This was remarkable because Schleicher had originally come to Texas with a band of followers in order to set up a communist colony, at the urging of his old friends Friedrich Engels and Karl Marx, the founders of communism. When the Texas community was on the verge of starvation, as everyone wanted to be a poet and no one wanted to be a farmer, Schleicher and his friends became born-again conservatives.

Due to a notorious incident during the ensuing war, known as the Nueces Massacre, the Texas-Germans, who constituted almost a third of the population of Texas, received a reputation for being pro-Union. However, they had voted overwhelmingly for Breckinridge and for secession, and later supplied, proportionately, more volunteers to the Confederate army than any other ethnic group, including the "Anglo" Texans. Many Germans fought under Confederate Colonel and (Provisional) General August Buechel until he was killed at the Battle of Pleasant Hill, Louisiana, and under Col. Gustav Hoffmann, a former Prussian officer and the mayor of New Braunfels when that German town was the third-largest city in Texas.

The procedures of democracy (if not always its substance) were sacred to Texans, and the issue of secession was put to the voters. The *Trinity Advocate,* the only newspaper in Anderson County, militantly supported leaving the Union. Texans arrived at their polling places in droves to decide the matter. The county remained united. A total of 870 voters, or 98%, voted to secede immediately from the United States, and only fifteen people voted to remain in the Union, at least temporarily.

William Howard Lawrence had named his only son, the author of this ledger, after John C. Calhoun, the philosopher and advocate of states' rights and secession. During the referendum, W.H. Lawrence addressed many meetings, giving passionate speeches for secession. When the war began, he was immediately elected colonel of the Home Guards. His age, and, one suspects, his prosperous girth, probably prevented more active service in the war, though there is oral history that he served briefly with the other Anderson County volunteers in Hood's Texas Brigade under Robert E. Lee in Virginia.

To modern Americans, secession from the U.S. appears drastic in the extreme, if not impossible. But at the time, Southerners were aware that some form of secession had occurred twice previously in America: At the Hartford Convention, New England seceded in protest against the War of 1812, and in 1833 South Carolina nullified all U.S. laws in protest against a protective tariff. Southern newspapers reported that Norway had peacefully seceded from Sweden only months before the South took that action, and several Southern states had already seceded before the Texas vote. U.S. President Buchanan had confirmed that the Constitution gave him no power to prevent secession—the matter was up to the states.

President Lincoln took no overtly hostile action until South Carolina's Fort Sumter was resupplied and thereafter fired upon. Then Lincoln called for 75,000 troops to quell secession. After the war, the prosecution of former Confederate President Jefferson Davis was dropped, out of a well-founded fear that the Supreme Court would reverse any conviction and openly declare secession constitutional and legal, despite the bloody war fought by the U.S. government to prevent it. The U.S.

Supreme Court had already ruled, in the "Prize Cases" of 1862, that neither Congress nor the president had power to declare war against any state or group of states.

Some modern Americans find it surprising that all classes of freemen in Texas, to greater or lesser degrees, supported secession, despite the known patriotism and loyal valor of the early Texans. What is often forgotten is that most Texans of the time had emigrated from the deep South, and in the schoolbooks of the time the American Republic was portrayed as almost exclusively the invention of the colony and state of Virginia and her heroes; therefore the South would be considered the legitimate heir of George Washington's legacy. (Hence his image on the Great Seal of the Confederacy.) They had immigrated into either the Republic of Texas or the Mexican state of Tejas y Coahuila. Their natural loyalty would then be to Texas or the South, not to a central federation of states. In the case of immigrants from elsewhere than the U.S. (a substantial minority), many had consciously chosen the Republic of Texas precisely because they had not wished to live in the United States.

Louisiana and Mississippi, when they were new territories of the U.S., were similarly fertile areas for Aaron Burr's secessionist fantasies in the early part of the nineteenth century. No oath of loyalty to the United States had ever been asked of Texans, though oaths to the Republic of Texas had previously been taken. Moreover, Texans had had the experience of a successful secession from the recently centralized government of Mexico, and of living in their own free, sovereign, and independent republic.

There was a small faction for remaining in the Union, led by the governor (and former president) of Texas, Sam Houston. Some of Houston's biographers speculate that he opposed secession in the hope of the future re-establishment of the Texas Republic. Others believe that he truly loved the American Federation that he had worked hard to make Texas a part of. Regardless, he was later loyal to the Confederacy, making numerous patriotic speeches for it and supporting his son in the latter's decision to be a Confederate officer.

Slavery was not as much an issue in Texas as in some other Southern states. There were far fewer black slaves, numerically and proportionately, in Texas than in the deep South. During the Texas Revolution, slavery had not been a serious issue despite the official opposition of the Mexican government to the institution. Cotton, the most labor-intensive agricultural product, was limited to specific areas of East and Central Texas, not expanding to the west until irrigation became common in the Texas Panhandle. Most slaves, therefore, were personal servants, rather than large, faceless masses of "field negroes." Under these circumstances, friendships and mutual loyalty did develop between master and slave, contrary to the unceasingly resentful relationships portrayed in modern books and movies. Many of these friendships continued long after abolition. Slavery was also less onerous in Texas because independent-minded African-Americans could more easily escape: Texas had virtually no slave patrols ("patterollers") to retrieve them, nor were the fugitive slave laws, enforced in the Northern states, of any effect in West Texas, Indian Territory, or Mexico. Texas slaveowners had to ensure at least somewhat more humane treatment than in some parts of the Union, and manumission was more common. Owing to all of these factors, Texans, on the whole, did not feel as seriously threatened by the issue of slavery.

Among Texans, secession from the U.S., as from Mexico, was more an abstract sentiment for local rule, local loyalties, and theoretical (or constitutional) liberty as displayed on the Alamo flag. The flag was emblazoned with "1824," the date of the Mexican Constitution, which many Texans claimed to be fighting for in that war. In other words, states' rights was their issue. This is not to debate revisionist historians who have proclaimed the slave issue as the major cause of the War Between the States (even if secretly or subconsciously) but to bring needed attention to the particularity of Texas and the motivations of its people.

Despite this, there can be no doubt that abolitionism itself was considered abhorrent in Texas, and not just as a reaction to "Northern meddling" (though that caused the outspoken defense of slavery). Texans possessed a sincere fear of both the social and economic results if slavery were abruptly abolished— fears which were justified, to some extent, during Reconstruction. Although Abraham Lincoln consistently denied being an abolitionist, doubts on this score, concerning a newly elected "centralizer," combined with the secession of other Southern states, was enough to provide the final push in Texas.

Whether secession from the U.S. was wise is, of course, a different matter entirely. Suffice it to say that to a lot of Texans, it seemed like a good idea at the time.

These historical events, and the war itself, were a well-remembered part of W. J. C. Lawrence's boyhood and youth.

When President Lincoln called for troops to suppress the South and the conflict was joined, Anderson County responded to its new nation. Over a thousand young men volunteered for cavalry and infantry regiments, most of whom fought with General Hood in the East. Anderson County's John H. Reagan achieved distinction as the only member of Confederate President Davis' Cabinet who served in the same position (postmaster general) throughout the war. The only other famous contemporary "son" of the county was the great chief of the Comanches, Quanah Parker, born to Cynthia Ann Parker, who had been abducted as a child during an early Indian raid against the leading frontier family in the area. The extended Parker and Lawrence families were close friends.

Colonel Lawrence was active in the mobilization and supply effort for the War Between the States. Commander of Home Guards was not as insignificant a position as it would now be considered. Texas was invaded five times (never successfully), and fifteen battles or skirmishes were fought in the state and on its New Mexico-Arizona border, including the important Confederate victories at Sabine Pass and Galveston. The last land battle of the war was Palmito Ranch, near Brownsville (it, too, was a Confederate victory). Much of the cotton raised in Anderson and neighboring counties was smuggled through Mexico, to be traded for guns and equipment for the Confederacy. Some of the bales were used as armor for the "cotton-clad" gunships that helped win the Battle of Galveston. Anderson County was also actively engaged in the manufacture of military supplies, and growing food for the Confederate armies.

Colonel Lawrence and his teenage son, Calhoun, participated in all of these endeavors.

Two large, colored tintypes in an elaborate gold-leafed frame of the period still exist of William Howard Lawrence and

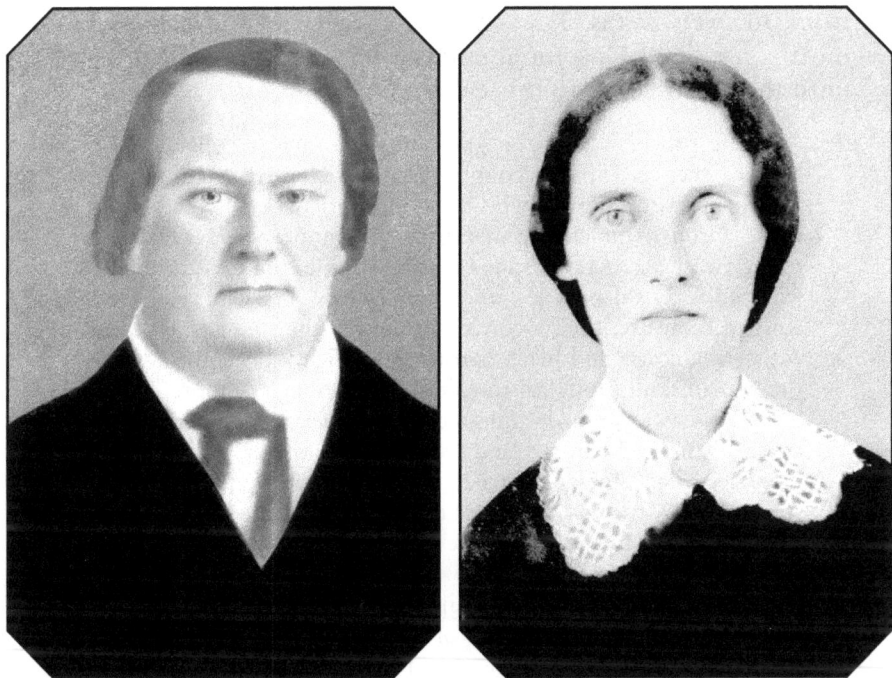

William Howard Lawrence and his wife, Clarissa Moody Givens Lawrence.
— Photos courtesy of Jane Day Rambie

his wife, Clarissa Moody Givens Lawrence, taken about the time of the war. Colonel Lawrence is shown in a black frock coat, fold-over collar, and black string tie. His hair, still dark, is longish and covers most of the ear—a style no longer fashionable at that time. His nose is straight but appears somewhat pugnacious; his mouth is similarly straight, in a typical Victorian unsmiling pose. He has gray or blue eyes. His jowls are heavy, leaving him with little suggestion of a neck.

Similarly, his blue-eyed wife is in a typical pose of the period: dark hair divided in the middle and pulled back in a bun; nose straight; white lace collar, closed with a brooch or locket. She appears slender but womanly.

Col. William Howard Lawrence died December 6, 1871. His funeral was delayed for five months because the ground was frozen too hard for speedy digging, and, some delay being inevitable, the family desired travel time for Masons coming from all over Texas. Lawrence later received the largest and most ceremonial Masonic memorial service ever seen in Texas until then, according to the *Trinity News (Advocate)*:

> The procession to the grave was the largest collection of Masons ever seen in this county. First came nearly one hundred and fifty Master Masons with their appropriate devices, and with white aprons, emblematic of Purity and Innocence. Next came thirty-two Royal Arch Masons with the Ark of the Covenant and with red aprons denoting Fervency and Zeal. Then came eighteen Knight Templars, their swords gleaming in the sun, and clothed with black scarfs and black aprons, on which were embroidered the human skull (in italics amenio mori), emblem of mortality.
>
> Col. Lawrence had requested that the services be performed by the Knight Templars, and at the grave, which was partially reopened. They formed a triangle: and around them the Royal Arch Masons formed their circle; and still outside of them the Master Masons formed their lines as guard and foundation of the order.
>
> The ceremonies were beautiful and solemn and were impressively delivered by the proper office, inculcating fully the doctrines of the Christian Religion, and enjoining on the members a full faith in the atonement of the Immaculate Jesus.

The ceremony was arranged by Dr. J. A. Lawrence, Colonel Lawrence's brother, and Eminent Commander of the Knights Templar.

II.

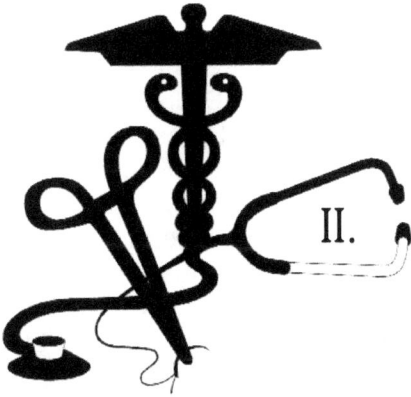

Medicine and Superstition

Young William Joseph Calhoun Lawrence, known as "Calhoun" in his family, was born in 1850. He grew up first with the hardships of frontier life, then the luxury, status, and privilege due a prominent family, followed by the work and alarums of war, followed in turn by the extreme privations and oppression of Reconstruction—all before going to college.

At the height of his prosperity, Col. W. H. Lawrence had owned black slaves. According to the census of 1850, he had three young male workers. By 1860, just before the war, he had eight slaves of both sexes on his large plantation, ranging from a ninety-year-old woman to a baby boy. He also had hired fieldhands. Lawrence's brother, Dr. J. A. Lawrence, owned thirteen slaves in the county. Large "slave-breeding" plantations were rare, if not nonexistent, in Texas.

Some would say that the Lawrence family, due to their slaveowning, "deserved" the bad times of Reconstruction. A mitigating factor on the part of Colonel Lawrence might be his policy of requiring Christian matrimony among his cohabitating slave couples in order to hold families together, rather than the more common policy of discouraging or forbidding marriage for fear it would complicate further sales of slave family members. However, the idea that those who had prospered by living in a slave-owning society deserved their fate would have condemned almost all Unionists from Missouri, Kentucky, West Virginia, Maryland, Delaware, and Washington, D.C. (Not to dwell on all of the other states in the early Republic, especially New England, much of whose wealth was based on the slave trade; also, all Romans, Greeks, Jews, Arabs, and Africans, and several other nations as late as the end of the nineteenth century.) Indeed, major Unionist heroes also directly profited from their slaves, including President Lincoln (whose wife was such an owner), General Grant, numerous members of the U.S. Congress during the war, and arguably the best general of the Union side, George Henry Thomas of Virginia, "The Rock of Chickamauga." By contrast, Robert E. Lee freed all of the slaves he inherited, both originally and through his wife, and devoted years, taking leave of absence from the army at no pay, to finding them remunerative employment. Also, the General Assembly of Virginia came within one vote of abolishing slavery before the war.

By the time Calhoun was sixteen years old, food was scarce, employment nonexistent, land titles fluid, taxes confiscatory, and society in turmoil. When he reached his majority, he was forbidden to vote or hold office, as part of the "old order." Reconstruction in Texas was the longest and most restrictive of the entire South. The new governor, Edmund J. Davis, was elected only due to Federal control of the entire election process and disenfranchisement of almost all whites. Davis had been a secessionist candidate for the Texas Secession Convention, and, when he lost, turned bitterly against the Southern cause. He became a Union officer, and staged at least one (unsuccessful) invasion of Texas.

When he ran for reelection as governor in 1873, he lost, but refused to give up the office. Davis ruled the state as dictator, declaring martial law and leading the new state police on a reign of terror. He took upon himself the appointment of thousands of new state officials, leaving almost none to the voters.

Davis had never been able to establish a political base and had to rely on continual reinforcements of Northern troops and bayonets to stay in power. When Washington finally refused the governor's incessant demands, Davis barricaded himself in the attic of the State Capitol in Austin and had to be arrested by the

Travis County sheriff and a mob of armed citizens. But his friends remained rich through corruption, while other Texans considered themselves lucky to eat.

As a reaction, the original Ku Klux Klan (first widely known as the "Knights of the White Camellia") was at its height toward the end of Reconstruction, numbering more members than had served in the Confederate army. Although myriad atrocities against newly freed African Americans were committed by the Klan, its original purpose, which it continued to adhere to and even accomplished to a large degree, was to protect wounded war veterans, widows, and orphans, and make life so difficult for the occupation governments and politicians that they would lose enthusiasm for maintaining Reconstruction. There is no evidence that any of the Lawrence family was in the Klan, nor was Anderson County a hotbed of that organization, but perhaps it is no coincidence that the most massively attended displays, ceremonies, and costumed parades of the Masonic orders occurred during the heyday of the first Ku Klux Klan. It is conceivable that Col. William Howard Lawrence's elaborate memorial service was such a pretext, though the fact, if true, would not have reflected on the family itself. Regardless, the original Klan was abolished in 1874 by former Confederate General Nathan Bedford Forrest, the reputed founder of the organization.

Revisionist historians have devoted books to the beneficial aspects of Reconstruction, and there is little doubt that some aspects, particularly the 13th, 14th, and 15th Amendments to the Constitution, benefited African Americans. Benefits to other people in Anderson County, or Texas, or to the application of the U.S. Constitution as a whole would be difficult to substantiate.

Under these unsettled conditions, Calhoun managed to attend the Medical College of Missouri at St. Louis, receiving his doctorate of medicine on March 4, 1875. He returned to Anderson County, Texas, to set up practice, and eventually treated almost everyone who resided in the county, and most of those just passing through.

Dr. W. J. C. Lawrence was always visibly noticeable among his peers. He was often mentioned as having a strikingly handsome appearance (or "profile," as Victorians put it), with fierce

— Diploma courtesy of Jane Day Rambie

blue eyes, a straight nose, and wide mouth. His auburn hair was
so soft and wavy that both his wife and daughter were known to
have lamented that they had no daughter with such hair. In his
ambrotype with his mother, and his colored tintypes (page 17
and later), he wore his hair longish and piled behind the ears,
and his mouth was set firm. Perhaps his jaw, though manly and

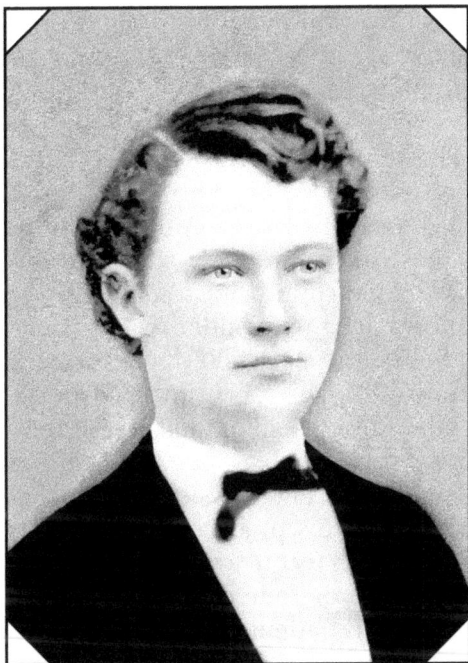

A young Dr. Lawrence.
— Photo courtesy of Jane Day Rambie

wide, was not as deep as he would have preferred, causing him to grow a mustache and goatee as soon as he reasonably could. His vanity was as well known as his appearance. It is possible that Lawrence would have been pleased to know that he would not live long enough to lose any of his auburn hair. Other characteristics often commented on were Calhoun's fierce pride, his perverse sense of humor, his sharp wit, and his chivalrous solicitude for women of all ages.

But Anderson County never knew what he really thought of his neighbors. None of his patients were aware that he kept records not only of their illnesses, treatments and payments, but of their habits, character (or lack thereof), idiosyncrasies, and scandals.

One can only guess at the tedious hours Lawrence spent between his new patients by examining the rococo penmanship in his ledger, embellished with ivy twining about each letter, attempts at medieval or Renaissance calligraphy, scattered cooking recipes, and complex doodling, examples of which appear in this book.

Dr. Lawrence didn't limit his art to penmanship; he also used different colors of ink to express various emotions and attitudes: brown or purple for narrative; green, red, and blue for emphasis, extreme disapproval, and extreme approval (or wherever the contrast was pleasing to the eye).

The flowery handwriting wasn't his only secret affectation. The purple prose, the wretched rhyming, and the geometric precision of his written tirades (inverted pyramids, hourglasses, varying sizes and shapes of typography, careful symmetry or intentional asymmetry) make his writing a delight for aesthetes as well as Freudians.

Due to the economic disaster of Reconstruction in Texas and the local, if long-term, post-cotton depression, few had cash and Dr. Lawrence was paid primarily by barter. Although in his ledger he listed his own services in woefully vague terms ("Treated wife," "Childbirth," "Medicined [sic] son," "hunting accident"), and specific diagnoses are rare or nonexistent in the ledger, there is no reason to believe he charged even as much as his contemporaries, and almost all of his work involved house calls. The great American myth of house-calling doctors is greatly exaggerated; most doctors, even in Texas, had offices, and observed business hours. Few Texans had physicians in attendance at childbirth, for example; in this practice Lawrence was somewhat exceptional. His invariable custom was to determine a cash fee (usually fifty cents to three or four dollars), and then come upon a barter equivalent for his patients' goods or services.

Livestock, produce, and labor were relatively plentiful and cheap, so the ledger shows fair dealing throughout, at least on Dr. Lawrence's part. Typical ratios were 300 bundles of fodder for $6; 20 bushels of corn for $10; bale of cotton for $30 (cumulative medical bill over a year); 16 boards for $8; two days' hauling for $5; half day's hunting by "self" for $1.25; cow & calf for $12.50. The system must have worked, for the majority of his patients requested Dr. Lawrence's services again and again, whether he wanted the patients or not.

A few of his long-term barter relationships were exceptionally cordial, and even touching, as in his entry for W. J. S. Beall and wife (see next page), who had managed to run up a bill of $103.

> I told Mr. Beall as we came from Palestine that I would take 13 Gals. of molasses and squear [sic] off with him. Mr. and Mrs. Beall have always made me the very best of neighbors, never want any better, they are like the pumpkin bread Good Enough for me!!!

Other barters were less felicitous. "Dickson G. Russell (Parkers son in law)" owed Lawrence $52.50, which "Rufus

130

W. J. D. Beall

1880   1879

1879 To Amt. of old a/c.	$95 00	Feb. 16	By Cash	$1
1880		Dec. 20	" 16.00 Boards @ 80¢	8
Feb. 20 To Visit & medicine "Lady"	2 00	" 21	" 13 lbs. Nailes @ 10¢	1
" 21 " 3 " " " "	2 50	" 23	" Two days hauling "Willie"	
" 22 " " " " "	2 50		1880	
" 23 " Cash for flour	1 50	Jan. 2 By ½ days hauling "Self"	1
To amt. from Page 63	$103 50	Feb. 12 " Cow & Calf	12
To Interest on amt. unpaid to date		" 25 " 1 days work Self & Willie	2
"Above from Page 63"		Apr. 22 " 7 head of Stock Cattle	4
		By amt. from Page 63	
Oct. 22 Visit & med. Eddie	2 50	"Above from Page 63"	
		By lard	
		" Butter, 6 pounds @	
I told Mr. Beall as we came from Palestine what		" ½ days hauling "Willie"	1
I would rather 3 Gals. of molasses and square off with him		1881	
Mr. & Mrs. Beall have always made me the very best of		Jan. 18 By 3 Gal. Syrup	
neighbors. never want any better. they are like the pumpkin			
bread good enough for me!!! J.H.C. Lawrence M.D.			
1881			
Oct. 12 To Visit & Med. Miss Harriet $2 50			
" for Mari married window Sash	2 00		
" " Pres. & Med. Miss Harriet	1 00		
Dec. 15 " Cash on 13 gal. Syrup	5 75		
	$11 25		
Mr. Beall owes me 13 gals. Syrup			

Oquinn [sic]" agreed to pay by September 1877. O'Quinn finally paid with:

> twenty five hundred feet of refused lumber, not worth any thing, scarcely to any one.

Lawrence then added that "Russell also has gone west."

In the case of other patients, the goods or services were never paid in any manner, allowing Lawrence to give vent to his anger in the ledger, as in his 1878 entry for one Thomas Holt:

> Tomias Holdit. And so Tomias does if he ever gets any money, old clothes, Corn, Cotton, Goobers, taters, beefsteers, horses, Cows & Calves, Cotton Seed, beefhides, fodder, Cow Skins, oats, hay, pork, bacon, chickens, turkeys, even Guinnies, Geese, or pigs, he Holdsit So tight you never can get it.
> Good Evening, Mr. Tomias Holdit.

In another entry, in 1879 (see next page), Dr. Lawrence displays his disgust by indulging in artistic embellishment of his lettering and writing his commentary in one of his beloved geometric designs. The patient was "I. G. Hamilton, *The biggest rascal for his sense out of jail.*" Lawrence himself settled the bill "By Killing a chicken eating Shoat that I could not keep away and out of the [Lawrence] yard," and by venting against both Hamilton and his son:

> I guess the shoat will pay off the $27.00 account as old
> Griffie is about as trifeling [sic] as one could find very
> [sic] in several days hard riding, unless the searchers
> should meet his lovely boy and hopeful Eric.
> Hopeful did I say? Yes, yes, hopeful of
> THE STATE PENITENTIARY.

What did Dr. Lawrence's patients get for their molasses, fodder, lumber, and shoats? Most of Lawrence's descriptions of his medical treatments are as scanty as his diagnoses, but those that are noted seem to be conventional medical practice for the doctor's time. Often home remedies and readily available medicinal ingredients were prescribed in detail so that the patient could maintain his own health longer with fewer visits, and the cost of specially ordered patent medicines was lessened. Some of the doctor's separately listed general "Prescriptions" sound

110

			$	
March	15	To Bacon lb. 6		
	20	" Bill of Lumber, 96/4 ft.	9	65
	22	" Cash for Bonnet Goods		00
Apr.	12	To 167 lb. of hams @ 12¢	20	12½
	"	" 86 " Sides " 8	6	88
	"	" 141 " Shoulders 7	9	87
Jun.	1	" Cow & Calf W. B. Smith	13	"
Aug.	16	To Medicines &c.	10	00
Nov.	12	" Glass lights		65
Dec.	18	" 4 # of Coffee	1	00
			3	1¼
		To Plaster of Paris	3	
		from J. P. Coly	11	85
		To Cash on settlement	88	00

1880

March	12	To Cash borrowed for 3 weeks	$15	00

1881

Jan.	8	To Accouchement Mary and attention for three nights & two days	$25	00
Apr.	12	To order from G. W. Wilcox	2	00

March	15	By Bacon 6 @ 8 Linseed oil		
Nov.	16	By Board self and wife		

1880.

June	20	Settled with Ira Hamilton

1881

Apr.	2	By Cash	$15

1881

Apr.	27	By killing a chicken eating wheat that I could not keep away and out of the yard that would weigh about 5 lbs.

Say: Geo. Geo.
hopeful
of
THE STATE PENITENTIARY.

strange to a layman now, and might not have met with general approval then. As an "Expectorant" he recommended a concoction including "cannabis, belladonna, and sanguinaria"; for coughs he recommended a candy of flaxseed, licorice, raisins, brown sugar, and ginger "to give a slight acid taste," and included a detailed recipe for producing it; for "Obstinate Diarrhoea" he prescribed ipecac, salicin, and distilled spirits; for "Obstinate Constipation," plain white soap played a prominent part.

Two of Dr. Lawrence's prescriptions, given to a "Mr. Thrasher near Parson Artists" are intriging and, if effective, would be well received today. On May 16, 1880, Lawrence prescribed two medicines: one for "Insanity, Bad" and another for "Inebriancy."

In his ledger and in other writings, Dr. Lawrence left a rather full description of the general state of health and disease in East Texas in the 1870s. He gave a list, in order of most common occurrence, of medical problems he encountered. Using his numbering:

(1) "Clay-Eating Children." Many East Texans had come from Georgia in the wake of Sherman's desolation, where there had been a long practice, indulged in by the poorer white children as well as blacks, of eating red Georgia clay by the handful. Whether this met some exotic nutritional need, or was simply a way of filling empty bellies, was unknown, but it continued in Texas, where people had to search ravines and hillsides for veins of red clay without grit, stones, or black dirt.

(2) Malaria, and (3) "Black Jaundice." Dr. Lawrence correctly concluded that black jaundice, or "Black Fever," was merely a more virulent stage of malaria. It wasn't until the year 1900 that malaria, like yellow fever, was discovered to be caused only by bites from certain mosquitoes; until then the general consensus of opinion was that the disease was caused by noxious gases (miasma) from the decaying organic matter in swamps, and spread by human contact. Therefore, although quinine was prescribed heavily, the emphasis was on quarantining patients and sometimes entire towns. The symptoms of malaria were easily confused with many other fevers, such as typhoid, yellow fever, and sometimes even pneumonia, so quinine was prescribed for those diseases as well. Aspirin was not developed until the 1890s.

Dr. Lawrence advised his patients to avoid clearing and building on low ground and creek bottoms. He noted that when morning fog covered the valleys, the older people got sick and complained. But Lawrence did not believe malaria was communicable, and never recommended quarantines. Dr. Lawrence estimated that of those who contracted malaria and black jaundice or (4) yellow jaundice (yellow fever), only one in ten survived. There was no known cure for yellow fever, but many homeopathic and patent medicines often eased its symptoms.

After malaria and yellow fever, Dr. Lawrence's most common encounters were with (5) typhoid, (6) pneumonia, (7) dysentery, again due to eating habits, (8) cholera, which he noted occurred most commonly among children of teething age, (9) appendicitis or "bilious cramp colic," (10) broken bones, (11) teeth needing pulling—there being no dentist in his county, Dr. Lawrence had to fill this need—and (12) skin eruptions.

Although Dr. Lawrence served as the major midwife in his county, he saw no reason to dwell on that, since he did not consider childbirth a disease. But his disgust with the superstitions surrounding the process gave vent to his most acerbic social comments. With the economic decline, and therefore the decline of education, all the old "superstitions and false modesty" came back with a vengeance. Axes were put under beds to control after-pains and hemorrhage; "conversations with witches" became common again, and bedclothes would not be changed for ten days after childbirth, nor would any water be used. One custom met with Lawrence's approval: No woman was left alone until the baby was one month old.

Dr. Lawrence noticed the increase of cancer, and predicted that one day "more will die from it than heart failure."

Still, with little contact or interaction among physicians, people "died like sheep." Out of five girl graduates of the high school in Palestine, four died by September. Lawrence was aware that the newer generations "did not die from the same thing one's great-grandfather did. New diseases make their appearance, old diseases succumb to modern remedies, and perennials have their ebb and flow."

There being no medical schools in Texas at the time Dr. Lawrence practiced, most other doctors had merely "read" medicine, by studying under a practicing physician ("preceptor"), after which they hung out their shingles. Although many became very fine physicians, this system led to varied schools of thought, with the resultant mutual antipathy, in addition to some quackery. Sylvia Van Voast Ferris and Eleanor Sellers Hoppe, in their fine study on early Texas doctors, *Scalpels and Sabres,* catalogue the various "sects," listing "allopaths, Thomsonians, homeopaths, eclectics, hydropaths, neo-Thomsonians," and others. This led to the clause in the Texas Constitution of 1876 that forbids the State to give preference to any school of medical thought or practice over any others, a proscription which is still observed. Most prominent physicians, like Dr. Lawrence, were "allopaths."

A common cure-all, to which Lawrence did not subscribe, was called the "heroic" method: "Bleed, puke, and purge." Emetics were tartar, ipecac, saltpeter, and opium, for vomiting and sweating, and calomel, castor oil, and mercury, for purging. Calomel had such drastic side effects that it was gradually discontinued. Topical bleeding actually did some good in snakebite cases, if only by accident. (The sucking of snakebites was a Hollywood invention.)

Arsenic and strychnine, in small doses, were mistakenly believed to stimulate the heart.

Ferris and Hoppe give a disturbingly thorough description of the prevalence of alcohol, usually in the form of whiskey or brandy, as a "tonic." It was considered a stimulant to the "mucous membranes of the stomach as well as to the heart," a general remedy for snakebite, and a germicide when taken internally. It became even more popular after the discovery of bacteria, and was given in large doses for diphtheria. Liquor was prescribed for typhoid, pneumonia, and diphtheria, even in children. The recommended dosage "was large enough to produce considerable intoxication on the part of the patient." Ferris and Hoppe report that "some physicians even considered the temperance movement a threat to medicine and health." Dr. Lawrence did not agree, being a teetotaler.

The most common painkillers were opium, morphine, and cocaine. The addictive effects of opium and morphium went unnoticed, and in one small town the entire population became

addicted. Deaths due to self-administered overdoses were attributed to "opium poisoning," and as more of these occurred, doctors changed to cocaine. Only at the end of the nineteenth century did drug addiction receive recognition as a social and medical problem.

The particularity of Texas was noted by Ferris and Hoppe in
the local popularity of Dr. J. Cam Massie's *Treatise on the Eclectic
Southern Practice of Medicine* (1854): "The work shows the rise of
states' rights medicine. Those living in the South believed that
there were certain differences [in their] diseases."

These interesting if idiosyncratic differences between nine-
teenth-century Texas medical practice and modern medicine,
which is usually considered the final word on scientific develop-
ment, provide an unfair view of early Texas. Medical discoveries
in the East and in Europe were assimilated as rapidly as possible.
Texas physicians quickly adopted inoculation (with syringes);
antiseptics; various successful surgical procedures and tech-
niques; effects of climate on respiratory diseases; the treatment
of wounds; and medicines and palliatives from quinine to ether.
More importantly, doctors took their psychological role more
seriously than some modern technicians. They knew their patients and they cared, and this caring showed, healing many a
usually lethal, if sometimes "only" psychosomatic, disease or
injury.

Despite all their misconceptions, early Texas doctors did
their best, under difficult circumstances. In his introduction to
Ferris and Hoppe's book, Dr. William M. Crawford wrote,
"During this period communications were slow and the inge-
nious Texas physicians devised many of their treatments by trial
and error. . . . These pioneer physicians were brave, bold, bril-
liant, and self-sufficient."

Not long after Dr. Lawrence began his circuit-riding medical practice, he opened a satellite office in Palestine, over a
drugstore. Soon he found a partner, J. F. Cely, a "Superinten-
dent" of the Southern Methodist Conference, and bought out
the lower store, naming it, grandly, "Office of Lawrence and
Cely, Staple and Fancy Groceries, Dry Goods, Hardware,
Queensware, and Drugs," with his and Mr. Cely's names en-
graved at the top of the stationery. This store would become a

great boon when Lawrence finally married and began a family. But until then it mainly served as a liquor store. Perhaps he was able to purchase spirits at a discount or tax-free, being a physician.

The account of 1877 consists almost entirely of daily sales of liquor (whiskey, gin, and bitters, by the quart and gallon) and tobacco.

Dr. Lawrence and Cely may have been teetotaling Southern Methodists, but their customers certainly were not.

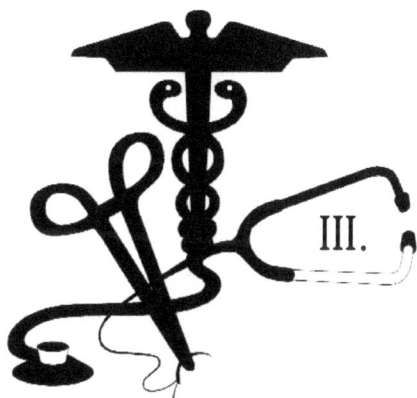

III.

Deadbeats

Despite all the bartering for services, some of W. J. C. Lawrence's patients had to be charged cash. One page of recapitulation is ecstatically entitled "Cash! Cash!" Collection was difficult when one lived in a waystation for points farther west, and during hard times had to treat all persons in need of medical help. Though Dr. Lawrence appears never to have actually turned down a patient (though he threatened to do so in the future, in several entries), he was not shy about attempting to collect his fees afterwards, or writing down his frustration and fury when he failed.

Many he wrote off without much further thought, such as William Sowell (treated from 1878 to 1881):

> By the help of God and my close attention to him, I saved his life but he never appreciated my services at least he went off without so much as thanking me. Shame on such a man.

Or Nathan G. Dunlap (1877-1878):

> Placed on the Dead head list—Get all he can and pay as little as possible, if anything.

Or "James Gentry (at Tom Mopes)," 1878:

> Run away and I guess that ends it, as far as pay.

One wonders if some of these were "Yankee Carpetbaggers"

69

Nathan, G. Dunlap.

1877				1878			
Oct.	31	To Visit & med Child	$7 50	June 20	By Cash in full	$7	50

1878

Aug						
Aug	29	To Pre & Med Baby	$1	50	Placed on the Dead head
"	30	" Visit & med, "	2	50	list; get all he can and pay
Sept	3	" " " "	2	50	as little as possible, if anything

1878		**James, Gentry**	("At Pine Hopes,")		
Feb	13	To Visit & med Self	$3	50	Run away and I guess
"	14	" Cash Visit & med,	3	50	that ends it, as far as pay
June	24	" Pre & Med Self	1	50	
July	12	" Dress "	3	50	
		1879			
Aug	8	To Visit and account Lady	12	50	
		1881			
Nov.	13	To Visit & accouchement Lady	12	50	
			$37	00	

on their way to the capital at Austin in the hope of still making their fortune from Reconstruction. If so, they were too late; it was over. The new Texas Constitution of 1876 (still in effect today, though frequently amended) was specifically designed to prevent recurrence of the abuses of the period of "Radical Reconstruction." Salaries for State employees were reduced, and written into the basic law; terms for public officials were shortened; most previously appointive offices were either abolished or made subject to election directly by the people; taxes became extremely difficult to increase; the powers of the governor were drastically reduced, making it impossible for him to act arbitrarily (or, to some extent, even govern); property rights were fully protected; and Texas reasserted her sovereignty. Though some measure of prosperity returned to Texas, Dr. Lawrence's ledger still reflected his difficulty in collecting his fees.

Some debtors merited special attention by Dr. Lawrence, as did John L. Cantrell (1881):

> This Dogon [sic] reprobate never did intend to pay me although I attended him faithfully during an attack of dropsey when every person and the Drs all gave him out to die, but if I ever do again you may have a joint of my back bone for a soup bone. Blame such a way to have to credit off an indolent Scamps account.

Fate helped Lawrence get his revenge against W. Ira Hamilton, perhaps a relative of the "I. G. Hamilton" whose family, rascality, and shoat were commented on at length (see pages 20-21). Certainly the name "Ira" appears in the earlier entry in an ambiguous way. Lawrence subscribed under W. Ira's name (1879): "Fool," "Liar," and "Puppy," and then, in calligraphy reminiscent of a medieval illuminated manuscript (which compensated for his inexactitude of spelling) appended, "The Most Contemptable Fool, Schoundrel, Liar, and Thief in the neighborhood." Above the insults—maybe in expectation of a suit for defamation—Lawrence wrote, "I can substantiate the following assersions [sic], if necessary, *In Any Court*" (see page 30). It is possible that he was unaware that, in a court of law, the burden of proof shifts to the defendant to establish truth as a defense, and Lawrence's allegations are not amenable to objective proof. However, the matter soon became moot:

I had to make the dastardly *Puppy* believe his time was up, if he did not pony up, and [I] was not mistaken.

Other debts were settled by the Grim Reaper, as on December 21, 1879:

Charlie Cash died today and I guess that pays his account.

Dr. Lawrence sometimes went to great lengths to collect the fees owed him, as in the case of the $27.50 debt of one John Hines (1877). The first entry exhibits merely impotent rage at the vicissitudes of fortune:

Stole Cattle and was Sentenced to the Penitentiary and Escaped from custody. Had better hung the Scoundrel.

Lawrence appears to have detected the scoundrel's spoor in April 1881, when, after adding four years' interest, he records that

I sent his account to him in the Indian Nation by John Mose and Jim Gentrys wife.

Whether the fugitive was ever found, repented his past and paid for his doctor's services (if not for the stolen cattle)—or was killed by hostile Indians—is not recorded.

One of Dr. Lawrence's deadbeats ("Henry Curtis [chizel fist]") drove him to the extremity of bad poetry, as shown on page 32:

> Chizel fist Curtis is my name,
> Buncom, bouncing, pudding and tame,
> If you want any more just blow me a reel
> For I ain't fit to sit in lower 'Hades.'
>
> I came into this world with a chizeling fist,
> I've chizeled them all in rain, snow and mist
> I've chizeled my wife nigh out of her will.
> I've chizeled the Doctor smoothe out of his bill.

Lawrence then admitted,

> And the fact is true further than all that—he is a much greater success at chizeling than I am at being a rhymist.

Some of the poor in Anderson County received kinder mentions by Dr. Lawrence, though no fewer attempts to collect. One such was one Bill Sauney (1878), who owed $1.50:

> I do not know what has become of "Bill Sauney." I have not seen the Scamp for a long, long time. Bill is a bad one, I can tell you. If I ever see William I think I will try to influence him to settle the above. I refused at first to give him any medicine for as I told him I did not believe he would ever pay me but he promised he would. I found him down in the field, he was living that year with Harrison Dean the year he lived upon Old Man Michaums place, he was down in the field picking cotton and I went down there to see Harrison Dean.

One might look at Dr. Lawrence's handwriting above this entry (page 33) to see that his calligraphic display of the entire alphabet was only slightly more elaborate than his opinions.

In the entry on Daniel Donnell (1877) the doctor seemed to accept a cosigner.

195

Gurry Curtis (Chizel fist)

1878

July	16	To S.P. & First, Lady		$4	00	
"	17	" " " " "		4	00	
"	18	" " " " "		4	00	
"	19	" " " " "		4	00	
July	20	" Quinine & Visit "		4	00	
			$20	00		
		Interest 1879, 80, 81	6	00		
		off on new book				

Chizel fist Curtis is my name,
Buncomb, bouncing, pudding, & tam
If you want any more just blow and spue
"For daint fist to sit in lower "Hades"

I came into this world with a chiseling fist
I've chiseled them all in pain I now & miss
I've chiseled my wife nigh out of his own
I've chiseled the Doctor smooth out of his bill
    And the fact is true further than
all of that he is a much greater success at chiseling
than I am in being a rhinest.
            J.H.Q. Lawrence
Sept 25th 1880.

Arnick & Henry, Baywell, (at John Hallam's)

1878

June	25	To Visit & Consultation with Dr. R. R. K. Hartman for Henry Baywell.		$5	00	

Arnick, well I guess he is excusable
the poor fellow has been working, there he
never drew any wages, and of course he
could not pay his debts, Messrs
Ward, Dewey & Co, of Huntsville
should learn and if necessary be
forced to pay their employees more
and at regular periods this way of
keeping a man at work for the
from two years to his life time
and never saying a word about
a settlement financially only
at the end of their contract and
the poor fellows then even in
debt the old clothes all. Shame
and yet we satisfied very strange

204

1878   Ennett, Gregg   1878

1878					1878		
Oct. 24	Do Visit & Med. Self	$2 50		Nov 5	By Cash		$4
" 25	" " " "	2 50			1879		
Dec. 12	" " " "	4 00		Jan. 1	By Cash		10 00
" 13	" " " "	4 00		" Discount		3 "
" 14	" " " "	4 00				
		$17 00					$17 "

	1880				1880		
Sept. 17	Do Visit & Med. Self	$5 00		Nov. 2	By Cash		$10 00
"	" " " "	50					
		$11 00					$10 00

1878   Bill, Sawney, Junc,

Oct. 9 To Pre. & Med. Self $1 50

I do not know what has become of Bill Sawney. I have not seen the boy for a long long time. Billie's a bad one. I can tell you. If I ever see William I shall try to influence him to settle the above. I refused at first to give him any medicine on it but him I did not believe he would ever pay me but he promised he would. If down in the field he was living that year with Harrison Dean the year he lived upon Mr. Hugh McChanns place, he was down in the field picking cotton and I went down there to see Harrison Dean.

J. T. Wilson Laurens, M.D.

Dan, paid me his own note in full, and concluded he did not feel able to pay his Uncle Demsa Fosters acc. for his Grand Ma Foster, So I am satisfied any way for Dan is a good fellow and has been more unfortunate than I have. wish every body was as good as Dan Donnell. if they were we would have a good country, *I think.*

However, on the same date in the ledger entry of Demsa Foster, Lawrence wrote:

Never having said anything to Mr. Foster about the agreement Dan Donnell made to settle the above and as Dan does not feel able to spair [sic] the money except two and one half dollars *I will charge the remainder to Mr. Demsa Foster.*

A later entry indicates that Dan Donnell paid it after all.

Sometimes Dr. Lawrence's better nature and wit overcame what could easily have become just another vitriolic diatribe against a deadbeat, as in the entry on Aenic and Henry Bagwell ("at John Hallum's" 1878):

Aenick, well I guess he is excusable the poor fellow has been working where he never drew any wages, and of course he could not pay his debts.

Mssrs. Ward, Dewy and Co. of Huntsville should learn and if necessary be fourced [sic] to pay their employees more and at regular periods this way of keeping a man at work for them from two years to his lifetime and never saying a word about a settlement financially only at the end of their contract and the poor fellows then even give back the old clothes all stripes and get away Satisfied very strange very strange Indeed!

"Mssrs. Ward, Dewy and Co. of Huntsville" was, of course, the doctor's euphemism for the State Penitentiary.

At least one female patient's bill was written off with kindness. The account of a Mrs. Bryant, who Lawrence cared for in 1875 and 1876, running up an account of $23, was closed in 1878 with the almost lyrical benediction: "Gone where the woodbine twineth. Gone west of course. Joy go with her now and forever. W. J. C. Lawrence."

Someone who dealt honestly (in a businesslike manner) with Dr. Lawrence always got his due in the ledger; often rewarded with an essay on his decency, as did the 1880 entry on

I. R. Emerson (see page 36), revealing Lawrence's business philosophy:

> Old friend Read comes up to scratch every time. [H]e fills my idea of a strictly business man, pays his debts punctually and wishes others to do the same. Any man who strictly adheres to this principal [sic] has my hand and heart—and can get any thing else I have if he wishes it (except the old woman) I wish every man had Read Emersons principals [sic] at least in this respect. But I fear that the Old man is not longer for this vain world. [H]e deserves great credit: few men have ever lived at least in this country who were his equal in financiering [sic] and in business prognosis. Come to this Country poor, broken up, and on the *wing*. Settled on the bank of a sickly creek and with land not even an average he has worked, managed to accumulate a very pretty support for himself and family in his old age. I am satisfied he has paid more Dr. bills than any two men in the country and while a good many who were well off when he was dead poor, have lived out and lost he has accumulated. I like *old man Read*!!!

Lawrence was capable of the enthusiastic exuberance of a small boy at Christmas when he was actually paid. Whether this outlandish emotionalism might have been caused by an unexpected rebirth of his faith in humankind, or, alternatively, to some desperate financial difficulty in his own family, is unknown. One Dave A. Saunders was the recipient of the most striking entry (see page 37). In letters over a half-inch high, elaborately illuminated and running lengthwise along the entire ledger sheet, Lawrence prints:

D. A. SAUNDERS IS AN HONEST MAN!
HE PAID THIS, AND CAPPS ACCOUNT!

> By Settlement at Mound Prairie Jan. 12th 1881. Saunders paid his own, and A. M. Capp's accounts except two dollars and twenty cents which I gave him, and I consider him reliable and a trustworthy gentleman as far as I know. [signed] W. J. C. Lawrence.

Nevertheless, Dr. Lawrence was a product of his time and region. Travelers to the British colonies of North America had often commented that the Americans were the most litigious people on earth. An astounding proportion of America's

134

A. R. Emerson

1880   1880

Aug.	29	To Visit & Med. Horse & Brin"	$3	00	July 20	By Cash	$5 00
		" " and atten. night	3	00	Nov 5 " Cash		65 00
"	30	" two Visits & Med. H.O.	3	00			$70 00
	31	" " " " "Horse	3	00			
Sept	1	" " " " "	3	00			
	2	" " " " "	3	00			
"	3	" " " " "	3	00			
"	15	" Visit & Med. Night "Self	3	00			
"	16	" two Visits "	3	00			
"	"	" making pills "Brin"	2	50			
"	16	" Two Visits & Medicine "Read"	3	00			
	17	" " " attention night	3	00			
	18	" " " " "	3	00			
"	19	" " " " "	3	00			
"	20	" " " " "	3	00			
"	21	" " " " "	3	00			
"	22	" " " " "	3	00			
"	23	" " " " "	3	00			
"	24	" " " " "	3	00			
"	24	" Rubber Syringe "Self"	2	25			
"	25	" Visit & medicine "Read"	3	00			
"	26	" " Detention day & night	3	00			
"	27	" " " " "	3	00			
"	28	" " " " "	3	00			
			$70	25			$70 00
		---1881---					
Nov.	17	To Call Visit & med. "Self"	$2	00	June 1 By H.J Lumber		
"	18	" Visit & med. "	3	00			
"	19	" Call Visit & med. "	2	00			

Old friend Read comes up to the scratch every t[ime]
he fills my idea of a strictly business man, pa[ys]
his debts punctually and wishes others to do th[e]
same. Any man who strictly adheres to
this principle has my hand and heart
and can get any thing else I have if he
wishes it. (except the old woman) I wish ev[ery]
man had Read Emersons principals at lea[st]
in this respect. But I fear that the o[ld]
man is not much longer for this vain wor[ld]
he deserves great credit. few men have ever li[ved]
at least in this country who were his equa[l]
in financiering and his business prognosi[s]
Came to this Country poor, broken up and on the
wing, settled on the bank of a prickly creek an[d]
with land not even an average by has work[ed]
managed to accumulate a very pretty support f[or]
himself and family in his old age. I am satisf[ied]
he has paid more Dr bills than any two men in th[is]
country and while a great many who were well off a[t]
he was dead poor, have lived out and lost he has accumulat[ed]
A like old man Read !!!! *A. R. Emerson* $70 0[0]

                                        1881

125

Dave Saunders

1879   1880

Dec 24	To Tobacco	$1 00	Mar	By work in [?] to date $7 95
	" Coffee	1 00		
	1880			
Jan	To 43½ Bush corn @ 75¢	32 62½		
Jan 7	" Coffee	80		
"	" Salt one pound	X		
"	" 42 pounds of [?] 7¢	2 81		
" 8	" Visit from a [?] "Lady"	8 00		
"	" 1 Turning plow	75		
	" 1 Sweep	50		
	" 1 Bull tongue	50		
	" 1 Grass rod	35		
	" 1 Heel bolt	15		
	" 1 Hoe	70		
Mar 16	" Order [?] Mdse	29 25		
Apr 15	" " " Flour	2 15		
May 1	" " " Corn 10 bu	8 50		
	" Such Flour, salt	2 15		
Aug 19	" 50 pounds of bacon	6 25		
	" 12 % interest on a/c			
Dec 1	" Cash in Palestine	50		
	" Hauling 8 bales	8 00		
	" weighing 8 "	80		
	" bagging & ties for 8 bales	14 70		
	" Cash to Calhoun	69 10		

D. A. SAUNDERS IS AN HONEST MAN! HE PAID HIS AND CAPP'S ACCOUNT

[vertical handwritten note] By Settlement at Mound Prairie Jan. 12th 1881 Saunders paid two and [?] M. Capp's account except two dollars and twenty cents which I gave him, and I consider him [?] and [?] as good as I know. R.W. [?]

ISAAC HENRY.

1881				
Jan 21	To Visit [?] Med. & self & [?]	$10 00		
" 23	" " " " "	10 00		

"Founding Fathers" were lawyers, meeting the demand for their services. Moderns are wrong when they write of the "new" fascination with lawsuits (though not the unconscionable expense now involved). This ancient American obsession with legal processes has continued to the present day, but was common enough in the past that small towns throughout the South, in particular, often had "Court House" as part of their names. There might not have been any other structures in such "towns," but the judicial center was always essential, with the courtrooms crowding out other governmental or administrative space.

Any list of North-South battlefields in Virginia will include dozens of names like Chancellorsville Court House, Spottsylvania Court House, Appomattox Court House, etc. One would think the war was fought almost entirely by lawyers. For that matter, the number of former Confederate generals and other officers who died of gunshots during trials in which they were counsels is exceeded only by earlier battlefield casualties as a cause of premature demise within this class. Despite the fact that they were often not permitted to practice law during Reconstruction.

This litigious tradition can probably be traced to parts of rural England, where as late as the turn of the twentieth century a country squire would hardly consider himself usefully employed unless he had several lawsuits (usually boundary or poaching disputes) against his neighbors. Charles Dickens had delighted in portraying such characters.

In the allegedly hot-headed American South this appeal to the courts might seem strange, considering that duels were legal until at least 1818, and were regularly tolerated for decades thereafter, despite sporadic social as well as legal sanctions against the practice sometimes called in C. F. Eckhardt's memorable phrase, "pistols for two, coffee for one." Dueling survived long enough to be the origin of the famous shootouts of the "Wild West." (One prominent Texas lawyer—retired, of course —has advocated the re-legalization of duels, as less expensive and quicker than litigation, and equally likely to result in justice. His only cavil was, "Who's going to teach the Yankees to shoot straight so they'll stand a fair chance?")

Many saw litigation in court as though it was, as Clausewitz might have put it, an extension of the *Code Duello* by other means. Also, the public could enjoy the spectacle. Entertainment was scarce in many rural areas.

Dr. Lawrence, of course, took advantage of the tradition. First, he tried his own hand at law. On June 5, 1877, he tried to collect from "George House (lives at Wheelock, Robinson Co. Tex)":

> I sent the acc. to the Justice of Peace at Wheelock or to the constable there for collection also sent a note for him to sign if he did not pay it.

There is no indication whether the $50 owed was ever paid.

He soon acquired an attorney for collecting his fees from those who had property that could be executed upon and who had not "gone west" or to Indian Territory. According to his entry in the ledger he made an agreement with a Mr. James A. Emerson, Esq., to whom he

> brought such of these cases[,] not to charge any cash in these suits or to any others in which he failed to collect the judgment out of the other party. In other words not to charge me any cash for any business I had in his court. He agreed to this because I wrote up his tax rolls and done several other things for him and did not charge him for my services.

Lawrence used his attorney to collect a bill of $20.16 from Rev. M. G. ("Gabe") Elkins (1880):

> Settled by suing him and garnisheing [sic].

Assuming Lawrence used the right word, neither he nor his lawyer paid much attention to the new Texas Constitution, which forbade garnishing of wages. Reverend Gabe's own wife was willing to be Lawrence's witness:

> I will give Mrs. Elkins this for telling the truth in a suit I had against Old Gabe Elkins, her husband, her evidence in the suit caused me to get my money out of old Gabe.

There is a disproportionate number of patients in Dr. Lawrence's ledger who, like Elkins, are given the title "Rev." and who earned critical comments from him. This does not imply anti-clericalism on Lawrence's part. It is nearly impossible to determine which ones were actually ordained clergymen. At this point in Texas history an astonishing number of immigrants to Texas assumed the title, and there being several hundred Protestant denominations in the state it was not worth the trouble to establish their bona fides. A new arrival who did not have any visible means of support or any other claim to fame was often likely to declare himself a clergyman as a means of instant status among devout Bible-believers (especially since even imposters would have a working knowledge of lay preaching and the Holy Book themselves).

Titles had traditionally been admired and employed in the South. After the War Between the States, thousands of ex-Confederate officers and other former soldiers used them, especially since none of the honest claimants could have held official or retired status, and therefore had to rely upon past glory. But they all ran the risk of meeting former soldiers from their declared units who knew their actual rank, if any. Dr. Lawrence nevertheless recorded one John Young, whose title, captain, he doubtfully placed in quotation marks and underlined—twice. A similar means of verification applied to people claiming former political status. Only among the "Rev.'s" was there little chance of exposure.

Dr. Lawrence obeyed the courteous rule of using reasonable titles when addressing or referring to those who aspired to them. There is little indication that any of these titled gentlemen in the ledger had ever had a congregation.

Dr. Lawrence was also forced to use the law to collect from Rhube C. McFarline in 1879 (see next page):

> By Settlement I hope forever never again to have any dealings with him any way.

Dr. Lawrence records that he obtained a court judgment for $30 against one James Williams, who died in 1877. Lawrence seems to have gone through a series of changes of heart and soul-searching about the late Mr. Williams over the next five years. Whether this was caused by a profound respect for the memory of the dead, sporadic belief in the virtue of forgiveness, or whether it simply reflected Lawrence's whims, is unclear. Whichever the case, practicality won out in the end.

The first entry read, simply:

Jim is dead now, and I hope is in hell, son of a bitch.

The next entry, signed and dated January 1, 1878, shows no reconsideration caused by New Year's resolutions or otherwise:

Dead and perhaps in hell at least I hope so.

The entry signed and dated August 27, 1878, exhibits a surprising conversion in a man of such stubborn opinions:

> I will take it all back and hope & pray, he may have gone to heaven.

Some time later Lawrence begrudged his lapse, by adding an amendment (signed but undated):

> He *did* though, Steal $30.00/100 Thirty dollars from me and that he never repented of at least not enough to ever pay me. [H]e stole the money, caused by his own mean principals [sic] and assistance of Old John Prewitt & Dave Dickerson the two biggest hog thieves in Henderson County and that is saying a great deal.

A signed entry in 1882 (see next page), about the same long-dead patient, is somewhat hopeful (or merely wistful), and without further maledictions:

> Charlie Williams promised me he would dig or rather bore me a well for his brothers [acct]. I hope he will as I have never gotten any thing for waiting on him.

Dr. Lawrence appears to have been disappointed again, for in his entry dated January 31, 1883, he adds:

> It was last fall he promised to settle the [acct] as given above. George Caddo fmc brought me his note.

Collections on judgments have not improved in the 122 years since James Williams died. That Dr. Lawrence was largely successful at litigation might be attributable to the fact that one of his patients was Judge (and later State Senator) Alexander White Gregg.

Dr. Lawrence's large number of deadbeat patients does not seem to be due to overcharging for his services. Indeed, he seems to have undercharged. In their book on early Texas doctors, Ferris and Hoppe attempt to compare fees and incomes for practitioners in the nineteenth century. In 1838, forty years before Dr. Lawrence practiced, the Medical and Surgical Society of Houston agreed to a fee schedule which included: in-town house calls, $5 (double after 8:00 P.M.); out of town house calls, $1 extra per mile in daytime, and $2 extra per mile at night; advice and

Williams

Dead and perhaps in hell, at least I hope so.
Jan 1st 1878. W.J.C. Lawrence

Charlie Williams ... me he would die or rather bore me a note for his brothers a/c, I hope he ... as I have never gotten any ... for waiting on him,
W.J.C. Lawrence

... 31st 1883
It was last fall he promised to settle the a/c as given above, George ... brought me his note.

I will take it all back and ... pray, he may have gone to heaven
Aug 27th 1878. W.J.C. Lawrence

He did, though, steal $36.00 ... dollars from me, and that he never paid ... of at least not enough to ever pay me. he stole the money, caused by his own mean principals and assistance Old John Prewitt & Dave Dickerson the biggest hog thieves in Henderson Co and that is greatiled. W.J.C. Lawrence

Allen, Wm Smith, alias Watkins,

1876					1878			
Dec. 13	To Amt. of note		$4.	00	Oct 12	By Sellers assuming		$6 00
	" Interest @ 10 % 2 yrs.			80		" Deduction		
	1878							
Aug	18 To Dr. Mur Iron			1 50				
			$6	30				$6 00

Mrs Fannie M Lawrence

prescription at office, $5 (extra time, $3 per hour); delivering babies, $40 (difficult labor extra); house calls to several in the same family, $1 extra per patient for prescriptions; medicine furnished by physician, $.50 per dose; etc. The Society then noted, "Physicians were to present their accounts to the patient immediately . . .; if unable to pay, to sign a note for the amount."

Ferris and Hoppe then list a number of physicians in the next few decades, whose fees were comparable to the early fee schedule, until the 1890s, when physicians in Austin raised their fees somewhat, especially for in-office prescriptions ($2.50-$5); advice without examination ($1-$2); and setting of fractures ($10-$100). Communicable diseases cost fifty to two hundred percent more.

In marked contrast to both fee schedules, Dr. Lawrence's recorded fees in the 1870s and 1880s (omitting those paid by barter) show that he typically charged $2.50 to $3.50 for house calls spread over a county and a half, including medicine and dressing of wounds, no extra for nighttime visits or additional family members; opening abscesses, $1.50-$5; setting fractures, $10; office calls of all natures, $1; delivering babies, $10; tooth extraction, $1; and such medicines as quinine, morphine, iron tonic, and cough medicines, $.25 each.

Ferris and Hoppe report that the average annual income for physicians in early Texas was $500; at the end of the nineteenth century, it was still only about $1,000. For specifics, they give the average yearly income for doctors in the San Antonio area of the 1860s as follows: 1861, $400; 1862, $300; 1863, $1,200; 1865, $500; 1866, $600; 1867, $1,800 (in scrip). The two exceptionally profitable years can probably be explained by the presence of Confederate army barracks in 1863, and the new forts for the Federal Occupation Army in 1867. Although the military had its own surgeons, they were usually not medical doctors, but were instead trained to treat war wounds and other military injuries. Dependent wives and children commonly sought civilian doctors.

But Anderson County had no forts. At Dr. Lawrence's rates for providing medical services, his long hours of work and maintenance of a general store are understandable, as is his fury when his bills went unpaid by a "trifling, indolent scamp."

IV.

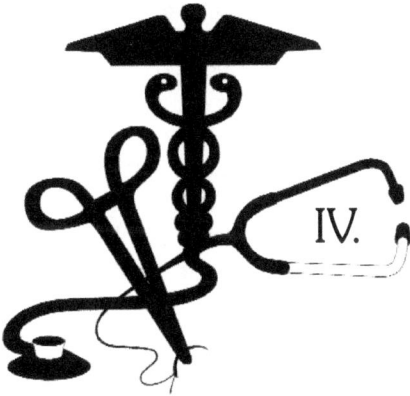

Family Values

The doodling in Dr. Lawrence's ledger diminished somewhat, and the denunciations became more acerbic when Dr. Lawrence added the responsibility of a family to his growing practice. After a long and ultra-proper engagement, he married Frances Mae Doss (June 2, 1862–April 30, 1940), a Georgian until the aftermath of Sherman's March drove her family west.

This background made her a match for her strong-willed husband-to-be. As a toddler in Conyers, Georgia, "Fannie Mae" had been told that the expected Union occupation soldiers were taking anything blue in color, so she sat for a day wearing her favorite blue dress covered by a large white duster, tugging on the hem of the latter to hide every glimpse of color. Her mother, Frances (Stansell) Doss, similarly had stood much of a day with one foot in a frying pan and the other in a pot, to keep the "Yankees" from taking them.

Fannie Mae went on to achieve local fame by shooting her father's jaw off when he returned home from Northern captivity in a borrowed Yankee uniform, a year or two after the war. Lt. Seaborn Peyton Doss (Company B, 18th Georgia Infantry) always remained inordinately proud of his little daughter's patriotism and marksmanship.

Fannie Mae was also remembered by her family for having complained bitterly to her parents, during the near-starvation of

45

Reconstruction, when meals were limited to sweet potatoes dipped in molasses, that her wicked brother "wiped his 'tater through the *middle* of the plate, and with the *big* end of the 'tater too!"

Fannie Mae was only fourteen when Calhoun met and fell in love with her, on June 24, 1877 (St. John's Day), as both of them meticulously recorded. Her young age, and her large, doting family would have insured the propriety of the courtship, even had Lawrence been tempted to be a cad.

The only surviving writings from Calhoun to Fannie Mae before the marriage are both on flower-embossed card paper. The first, dated August 22, 1877, says simply, "Miss Fannie Doss. Br. [Brother] Fowler preaches at the Camp Ground tonight. If you would like to go, and can condescend to go with me and wish to ride my pony, send me word, how about the company. Respectfully, W. J. C. Lawrence." The second, over two years later, was on the same type of embossed note card: "Miss Fanny Doss, Please accept my compliments, and if agreeable I would be pleased to escort you to the 'Foot washing' tomorrow." The Camp Ground was both a village and a Methodist revival meeting place.

Meanwhile, Lawrence was living at "Mrs. Hamilton's Boarding House," with two rooms. His family wealth and land having mostly dissolved during the war and Reconstruction, Lawrence had to plan a more spartan life for his future family. He built Fannie Mae a cabin near Camp Ground—two rooms and a kitchen with a big chimney. The walls were wood-panneled, tongue-and-groove, and painted cream. In those days, "building" a house did not mean hiring a contractor and picking out plans—it meant digging dirt, laying rocks, hammering nails, painting, etc.

Lawrence's first purchase was a cradle, followed soon by a room-sized rug, dark brown with big yellow flowers, considered the most opulent in the county. Lawrence also built a shed for his laboratory, which he later gave, rent-free, to an elderly black servant who had cared for Fannie Mae as an infant.

The wedding at the Camp Ground Church was November 16, 1879, a few days after Fannie Mae's sixteenth birthday (three weeks later Calhoun would be thirty). Although the entire population of the village and surrounding farms was only 3,000, at least that many came to the wedding, some traveling great distances and almost all bringing food for the feast.

Fannie Mae was considered beautiful, a blue-eyed strawberry blonde with a "creamy complexion and lips red as strawberries." The wedding tintype (next page) shows the Lawrences an impressive couple, in fashionable and well-tailored clothing. The picture displays the extra care with which he prepared his "wavy, auburn hair" and new mustache and goatee, with a wing-collar, four-in-hand tie and gold watchchain, and Fannie Mae's care with her trousseau and hairdress. Her mouth, slightly wider than the popular "rosebuds" of the period, was set in a soft, rounded chin which years later would form the basis for matronly jowls. (Calhoun would never, of course, suffer the ill effects of aging.) The couple was posed the usual Victorian way, with the lady standing to show her finery, and the gentleman seated, to keep their faces as closely as possible on the same level.

Everything seemed to go well until just after the wedding. On leaving the church the horse jumped its traces and tipped over the buggy. Lawrence was humiliated, exclaiming that "I thought I promised to protect you!" The couple returned to Mrs. Hamilton's Boarding House for dinner served by the landlady's freed slave, "Aunt Sarah Hamilton," only to be interrupted by a message from the family of a young woman who had gone into premature labor. Dr. Lawrence left after a few bites of food, and stayed away for three days. He returned still in his wedding clothes, which had been inadequately protected by a white linen duster. The battle for the young woman's life left him "tired, wilted, and soiled." Fannie Mae had considered visiting others during his absence, but the nearest neighbor (other than single male boarders) lived a mile and a half away, and she had no horse with her, so she stayed alone.

She never complained when her husband returned, thus receiving a reputation for courage and loyalty which Fannie Mae thought fraudulent, but she would not disabuse her husband.

Less than three days later, another medical emergency took the doctor away at 3:00 A.M. While putting away clothing when Lawrence was gone, Fannie Mae noticed a bulky weight in the white duster he had left behind this time. She reached in the big side-pocket and pulled out the deformed body of a still-born baby

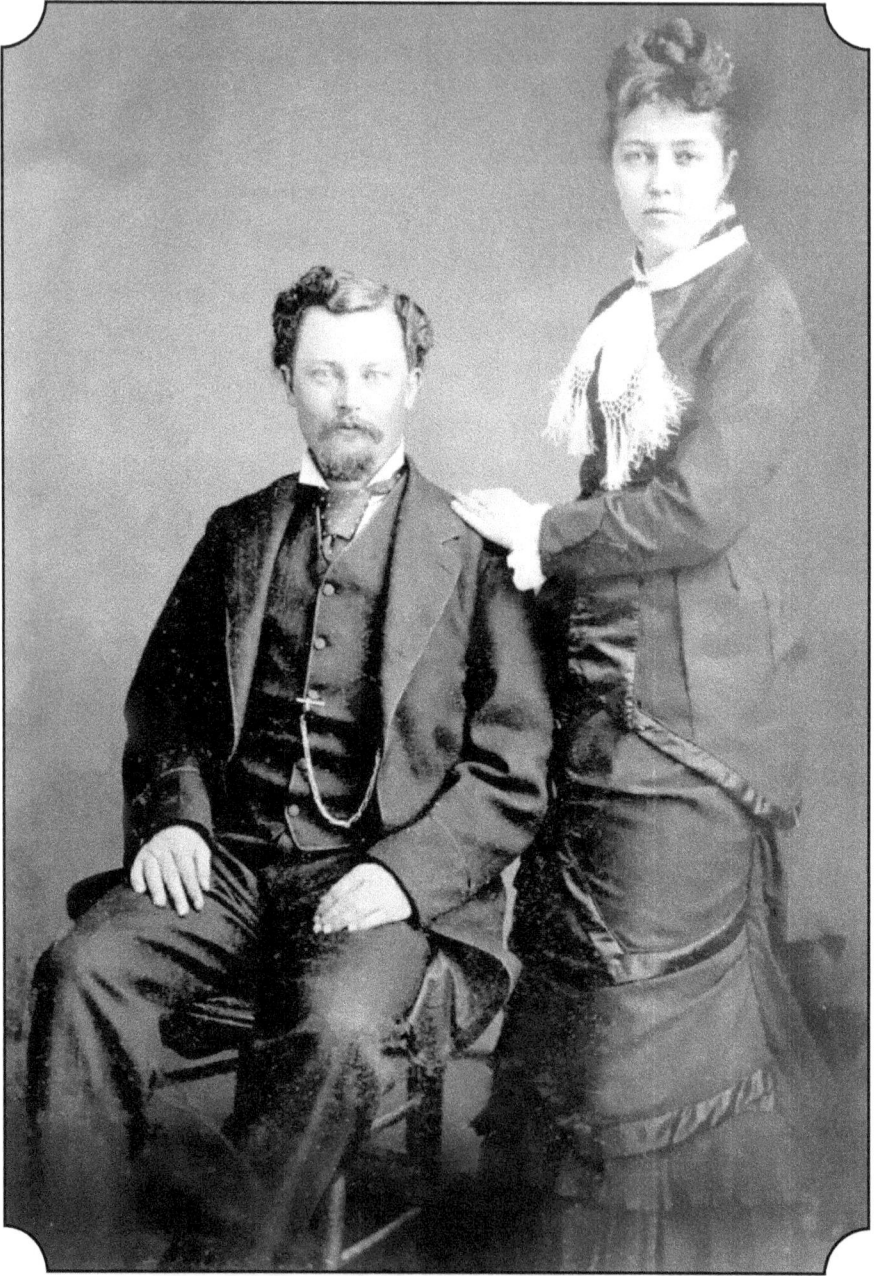

Dr. and Mrs. Lawrence
— Photo courtesy of Jane Day Rambie

which he had brought home to preserve in alcohol. This was too much for the young bride, and she ran away to her mother's house, cross-country and in the dark. It was two and a half miles away, so she arrived at daybreak. Three days later, Dr. Lawrence returned and brought Fannie's horse to her. His bride said she left due to loneliness, never mentioned the dead baby or her panic, and never endangered her husband's respect for her courage. Lawrence proceeded to immerse the decomposing corpse in alcohol.

Fannie Mae confessed in an interview in the 1930s that her fear during her husband's absences often caused her to spend the night hiding in her fig tree.

The couple lived at the boarding-house for a month, over the Christmas holidays. One of Lawrence's patients built them twenty-seven (!) chairs and two rockers, of white hickory wood, and they also managed to acquire a dresser, a chiffonier, a "turning mirror," and, finally, a bed, after which they moved into their new cabin. Fannie Mae was still proud of being married to "the most handsome man in the State" and being "a doctor's wife," and Lawrence was equally proud of Fannie's youth, beauty, and courage.

The barter system Dr. Lawrence had employed sometimes involved real estate transactions, and this helped him with his new family. In his ledger entries on Silas M. Parker, Dr. Lawrence recorded all treatments from 1876 to 1881. Many invoices during that period were paid with such items as "yoke of oxen" and "210 ft of lumber," but by 1881 there was still a balance of almost $100 owed to the doctor. On August 18 of that year, Lawrence records that he obtained $213\frac{1}{3}$ acres of land from Parker, at approximately $1.40 per acre, for a total of $300. This might reflect the low value of real estate at the time, or mean that Mr. Parker's previous debts to Lawrence were taken into consideration in negotiating the price. But the land could not have come at a better time, as far as his family was concerned.

Silas M. Parker had been the legal guardian of his sister, Cynthia Ann Parker, the mother of Comanche Chief Quanah Parker, after her recapture. She never readjusted to her native Anderson County and reputedly died of a broken heart in 1864. John Wayne's famous movie *The Searchers* was based (very loosely) on her story.

As late as May 1877 Dr. Lawrence must have still owned some of the land that had belonged to his father before the war, because according to his ledger he rented a portion of "my farm at Mound Prairie" for a $150 note from a Mr. Forbes. The plat for the rented land is sketched in the ledger and is notable for the fact that it was "surveyed" and partitioned only by the use of a length of rope which happened to be sixty-four feet long; all measurements (or metes and bounds) being based on the number of rope-lengths.

Dr. and Mrs. Lawrence proceeded, like other couples of their day, to have as many children as they could, as quickly as possible. And like other families, they were plagued by infant mortality. Erma Mary was born and died on July 7, 1881; Clarissa May was born on February 22, 1883, and died of measles at the age of nine, though she outlived her father. Leta Clementine, the only child to survive to adulthood, was born March 25, 1884.

Dr. Lawrence's desperation for a son, and Fannie Mae's love for her husband, might be inferred from the fact that their fourth daughter, born several months after Lawrence's death, was burdened with the name William Joseph Calhoun Lawrence. The infant died within a year of her birth. Whether her name hastened her demise is unknown.

(Dr. Lawrence's widow would later marry another physician, Dr. F. B. Moore, and name their daughter "John Ray"; two of Fannie's own sisters had been named "Willie" and "Vick." It is therefore likely that Fannie Mae enjoyed both life as a country doctor's wife and gender confusion in names. Perhaps having endured the Southern femininity of "Fannie Mae" all her life, she preferred masculine monikers.)

Dr. Lawrence's respect for his wife, for womanhood in general, as well as for his medical practice is reflected in the dozens of his letters which still remain. He apparently wrote to Fannie every day that he was away from home for even a few hours, either on his medical rounds or at his general store. Concerning his patients, childbirth and the health of the new mother were, to Lawrence, his greatest responsibility.

The letters exhibit none of the wit, sarcasm, or furious complaining so abundant in his ledger. Instead, his tone to her was always affectionate to the point of saccharine sentimentality. It must be assumed that Fannie Mae's formal education was somewhat limited, since Lawrence's extensive and exuberant vocabulary was reduced, in the letters, to only the most common and simple words. Of course, she was young enough to have received her only schooling during the hard times of Reconstruction.

On September 3, 1881, the doctor reported his extended stay with the wife of a Henry Henderson, who was having particular difficulties. "Had to spend night and couldn't sleep. Was very unwell throughout. Weak; threw up and run of the bowels all day yesterday without ceasing I was never much sicker in my life." He proposed a short vacation when he came home; he hated to spend the money, but Fannie was also pregnant, and "I would hate for either of us to die. I can not see how we are going to help it until we get better."

Lawrence was not guilty of the patriarchal sins often attributed to other Victorian husbands. In addition to building and maintaining the house, he took care of the children whenever he was home, cooked, washed, planned and planted Fannie Mae's kitchen garden, tended her flowerbeds, carried manure, etc. Both spouses referred to these activities approvingly and without indication of any imaginary "loss of masculinity."

For that matter, the entire concept of stern Victorian patriarchalism is undergoing re-evaluation. In the most extreme and persistent legend, a husband was legally permitted to beat his wife with a switch or stick "no thicker than his thumb." In truth, the earliest compilation of Common Law was William Blackstone's eighteenth-century *Commentaries on the Law of England,* in which there is a slighting mention of an "ancient" and long obsolete acceptance of wife-beating for "corrective" reasons (though no mention of a stick), and no court has since attempted to resurrect the idea. Wife-beating has always been illegal in each of the United States (two defendants claimed the "ancient law" in the nineteenth century, and lost). Wife-beating was not only held in extreme contempt and punished by the courts when discovered, but often led to public horse-whipping as well. Judging from his private writings, Dr. Lawrence would gladly have wielded the strap. Victorian pedestals for ladies, however, were very much in vogue, and Calhoun installed his wife on a marble one.

When away from home, Lawrence often explained his need

to "be a good sire and take good care of my old woman for I could not get along without her and if she was gone I would not come home." He excused himself again, on February 4, 1881, explaining that:

> I am fourced [sic] to be called away occasionally but try to make it as seldom as possible, *to secure You Some of the Comforts* of life and I must of necessity be called away from you once in a while, I have done very well so far. I collected twenty five Dollars yesterday and secured $15.50 more . . . Now 'Baby' dear take *especial good Care of yourself whenever I am away* and I can be happier and less uneasy for I can not help but be uneasy whenever I am away from you for fear you may be sick.

One letter written by the otherwise master stylist was not only sent the same day he left home on circuit but was solicitous to the point of incoherent babbling:

> . . . So please do not be uneasy at all, please baby, and I will bring you a nice present to make your purse heavier. [I will be home tomorrow] *so please do not be uneasy please.* [Visit Mrs. Beall if you are lonely] now baby please do not get uneasy and do as I ask for you know it is for the best or I would not ask it . . . If your Ma come [sic] get her to stay with you but if she will not go and stay with her. All will be right, dearest. Affectionately your devoted husband W. J. C. Lawrence.

To Dr. Lawrence, love must have meant always having to say you're sorry, for in a letter from his store written May 12, 1883, he apologizes that though he sent Fannie Mae six spools of thread, he could not find any pins—sold out—but "will keep a look out and send or bring them if I find them." He didn't find the sizes of needles she wanted, so he sent only one paper and would keep looking until he found another. He asks Fannie Mae for a longer list so he can show his devotion. He then sinks to babbling again:

> You requested me some days since to bring you some soap and really I forgot it every time I was at store and when I would get home I would think I will get it next time. So today I got it out as soon as I come to keep from forgetting, for I never fail to get what you request me unless I do forget it for I am shure [sic] you never ask for anything unless it is necessary but I cannot help forgetting sometimes let me try not ever so hard.

He also sent a bottle of shoe blacking "which does not require any rubbing to make a shine."

> Kiss little "baby May" for her Papa and tell her to kiss "Mama" twice for Papa. Please have Minerva to get me a bit of warm water so I can bathe after [I hope my customers] will be apt to turn out better late this evening at least I hope the Cash ones will.

Lawrence then asks his wife if she wants anything else, to send Minerva back down, and signs the letter, "Your affectionate old man."

While hunting for several days for his and Fannie's horses and a mule which had been chased off (presumably by one "Fred"), he kept his wife informed of his progress every few hours, by runner.

> Please tell Fred if you see him that I say him and Johnson had better get my horses up and if they [the horses] are hurt from their throwing rocks at them that they will find this a very unhealthy country for them, that as my horses are hurt so I put it to them that I intend to stamp Johnson and him if he had anything to do with the turning my horses outside much less abuseing [sic] them, and that [the horses] had better be up when I come and all right.

Lawrence found his mule miles away and it followed him home, but the fate of the horses or Fred and Johnson is unrecorded.

One letter which Lawrence wrote during an extended trip to Galveston displays the difficulty of travel at that time, the work of a part-time merchant, and the delight of a Texan's first introduction to electric lights:

> . . . 10:00 PM . . . I have arrived at the island City Safe and sound and as plucky as ever you saw me. I arrived at Palestine about 3 o'clock in the evening I left home, and the train for this place was due in Palestine at 11.50 that night—went over to Depot and had to wait until 4.20 in the morning. Came to Houston and had to layover, on account of being behind time until 3 in Evening. Came to Galveston and arrived here at 4.40 this evening, went arround [sic] and made the acquaintance of Legrease and Co, L.&H. Blum and went out to look arround

[sic] and take in some of the Town tonight. I was at an Auction and bought a few articles but nothing to amount to anything. . . . I bought Some Shears, one dozen vests, 4 sets of plate Silver forks and two plated butter knives. I am meeting with very warm receptions from the merchants here . . . in the morning I will finish Calling on the merchants and . . . will commence to buy my stock. . . . I bought . . . 4 knives and 4 money purses in Houston, think I got a bargain, cost 28 cts each . . .

Musquitoes [sic], Skeeters, Galanippers—I tell you have no idea I will get sleep tonight. . . . I tell you I could show you something to open wide your eyes. The electric lights are beautiful and are nearer that of the sun's rays and one light fills the place of half dozen oil lamps or more they are beautiful and are the first I ever saw. I am writing by the use of one now and can see everything like noon day.

Everything was up to date in Island City. However, Lawrence had discovered the attraction of electric lights to other life-forms, and hurriedly wrote that he must immediately turn out the light and "go to bed to keep of [sic] the Musquitoes, and cover up."

Family life did not temper Dr. Lawrence's vanity, as his wife complained that when he caught the mumps he would allow no one to know of it or see him, even from a distance, for the swelling that was "making such a grotesque caricature" of his handsome young face.

Dr. Lawrence's most vicious invectives against patients often clearly reflected his Victorian idolatry of womanhood (at least married womanhood—he usually ennobled a patient's wife with the title "Lady"). A typical entry denouncing a bad husband is that for his patient, one William Thompson ("William Mopes' Brother in law"), as seen on next page:

Of all the trifeling [sic], lazy, worthless, mean, insignificant, contemptable [sic], wife abuseing [sic], wife deserting, wife neglecting, diabolical Scamps who ever disgraced this Country and was the cause of so much trouble to a poor, inoffensive, downtrodden woman this "William" is certainly *the one*.

May the Good Lord take pity upon the world and save some person the trouble to kill him, for he is not worth killing the Cowardly, dastardly, poltroon.

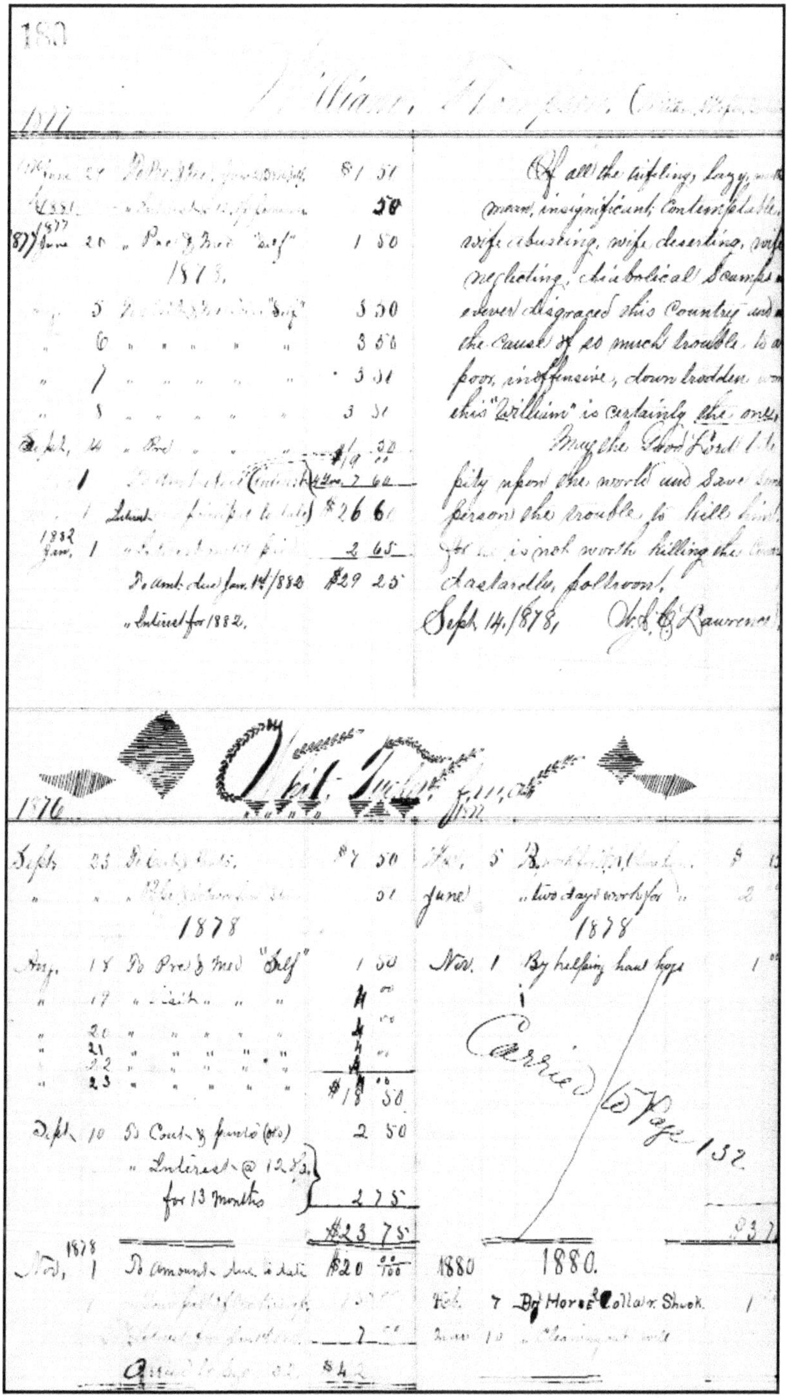

William Thompson

1877 June 20	" Pre & Med "Self"	1	50
1878			
Aug 5	" " "Self"	3	50
" 6	" " " " "	3	50
" 7	" " " " "	3	50
" 8	" " " " "	3	50
Sept 14	" "		
1882 Jan. 1		2	65
	To Amt. due Jan. 1st/1882	$29	25
	" Interest for 1882.		

Of all the trifling, lazy, ... mean, insignificant, Contemptable, wife abusing, wife deserting, wife neglecting, diabolical Scamps ... ever disgraced this Country and ... the cause of so much trouble to a poor, inoffensive, down trodden ... this "William" is certainly the one.

May the Good Lord ... pity upon the world and save some person the trouble to kill him, for he is not worth killing the cowardly poltroon!

Sept 14, 1878, W. J. C. Laurence

1876

Sept 23		$7	50	June	" two days work for "	2	
1878				1878			
Aug. 18	To Pre & Med "Self"	1	50	Nov. 1	By helping haul hogs	1	00
" 19	" Visit " " "	4	00				
" 20	" " " " "	4	00				
" 21	" " " " "	4	00				
" 22	" " " " "	4	00				
" 23	" " " " "	4	00				
		$18	50				
Sept 10	To Coat & pants (old)	2	50				
	" Interest @ 12% for 13 months	2	75				
		$23	75				
1878 Nov. 1	To amount due to date	$20	00/100	1880			
				Feb. 7	By Horse Collar Shuck	1	

Carried to Page 132

1880

As with all Dr. Lawrence's judgments, he carefully signed and dated this outburst (September 14, 1878), lest he, himself, be considered cowardly by his posterity.

Dr. Lawrence's affection for his own family is again revealed in a letter to his wife, dated 1884, which he wrote while on an extended medical emergency, addressed to "Darling and little Ducklings" and later attached by him to a page in his ledger. One of the "ducklings," Leta Clementine, took the liberty some time after her father's death to practice writing her name, as well as copying his penmanship, on several pages of Dr. Lawrence's "secret" ledger.

The only comment on his family's private life which Dr. Lawrence wrote directly into the ledger (see next page) was the last entry he made before his death, written in the account of a patient he had treated years before. It shows a gentle, comfortable familiarity that not all Victorian families achieved:

> I did not go to church today as I was so tired, not having had any rest for several weeks, therefore I prefered [sic] to remain at home as Jack Doss [an in-law] come up and he could take "Dear," in the buggy, and she would not be disappointed. I feel refreshed by my rest. Old woman will be home directly so I had better rest some more for she wont let me when she comes. She will want me to talk. God Bless my old woman. W. J. C. Lawrence.

Other people's families did not fare so well in Lawrence's estimation, though he was always careful to place the majority of the blame on the *paterfamilias*, as in his bitter epitaph for one David Woosley:

> Old David kicked the bucket and I guess he kicked so hard he did not leave any thing to pay an honest debt with, and if he did, the example of a non debt paying, ever avoiding an honest debt and an ill spent life in general has instilled fully into the minds of those he had influence over. The same base, mean, low down, trifeling [sic], lazy, low-lived principals [sic] inculcated within his own old mean breast.

Then comes the "prayer":

> May the Devil take a fancy to him for no one else ever could and he should have one friend.

206

1879　　　Wiley, Allen

Joseph Cullen Lawrence, M.D.

George, Jasper, June? 1879

Jack Rushing's family (who had run up a debt of $128) gets similar treatment in 1879:

> Old Jack has played out almost and for all the good he is to his Creditors or even to himself and family he had about as well be dead, for he never supported his children much less pay a debt. His oldest daughter works out for her living, and his boys from 12 years old and up to forty (for he has seven or eight) are tramping over the Country first here in this country and then out west but with the understanding always that they will not work. 'Spect I can guess what will becomes [sic] of them if they do not look sharp. The old Lady handed in her check two years ago next summer and I guess old Jack will hand in his this summer for when they get sick they generally die as they have treated every Physician as they have me and we let them play it alone.

Yet some sign of Lawrence's dispensation for the ladies shows through, however disguised, even in such a scathing attack as that on "Scown, Englishman at Mrs. Dan Millers":

> Old Scown is dead and his old wife ought to die also and go to womens hell if there is such a place.

The doctor's theological dispensation (if it can be called one) did not extend to those whom he considered "loose" women, such as "Mrs. Sophrona Devers (Mrs. Doughty's Niece)," who "Had a bastard young one and never paid for it." (See page 59.) Lawrence records that he later sent the bill (with three years' interest) to "her" father, F. M. Brown, never clarifying whether Brown was Mrs. Devers' progenitor, or that of the "bastard."

The " 'Widow' Porter" (1876) received only slightly greater sympathy, as seen on page 60:

> She, too, has taken Horace Greeleys advice and gone west. I hope she may do better there than she did here and not have any more "bouncing baby boys" without any "papa."

But then, she deserved kinder treatment: She appears to have paid her medical bills.

41

John Lawrence, Scarborough, Dr.

1877			1879		
	To Ballance on a/c, 1875	$1 00	Nov. 10	By Cash	$15 00
1878				" Discount	7 00
Jan 3	To Visit & Med. "Johnie"	3 00			
" 4	" " " "	3 00			
" 5	" " " "	3 00			
" 6	" " " "	3 00			
" 7	" " " "	3 00			
" 8	" " " "	3 00			
" 9	" " " "	3 00			
		$22 00			$22 00

Teta Lawrence

1878	Mrs Sophrona Devers, (Mr. Daughter)		Had a bastard young one and never paid for it.		
July 20	To Visit & accouchement	$12 50			
Aug 12	" Pov " Med Self	1 50			
" 23	" Open abscess "	2 50			
" 29	Visit atten. night "	3 50			
Sept 10	" " & Med. "	2 50			
" 14	" Pov " "	2 50			
" 20	" " " "	2 50			
		$27 50			

To Interest from 1879

I sent the a/c as above to D Mr Brown her
father with interest from Oct. 1st 1878 to
Aug 1st 1881 making 34 months @ 10% $7 56
     27 50
Aug 1st 1881 Rendered accordingly this date $35 06

174

"Widow" Dodd.

1876

To 5 Visits during the year	$17	50	
" family medicines	2	50	
" Interest to date one year	2	00	

1877

Feb 22 to 29 To visits &c from March 22 to March 29	24	50	
March 31 " med extra self & husband son	3	50	
Aug 10 " Visit & med self	2	50	
" " " " " "	5	00	
" 10 " " " "	2	50	

{ She, too, has taken Horace Greelys advice and gone west I hope
she may do better there than she did here and not have any more
"bouncing baby boys" without any "Papa".
                                                    H. G. Lawrence }

1877

Samuel Payne, f.m.c.

1877

Jan 6 To Visit & medicine "self"	1	50	June 9 By 12 bundles fodder		35
Apr 2 " " " " "	2	00	" Doctoring cow skins		25
Aug 18 " " " " "	1	50	1879		
" 19 " Salts "		25	Jan 6 By Cash	6	50
1878					
Dec 9 " Pres & med "	1	50			
1879					
Jan 25 To Visit & medicine Self	3	00			
	$9	75		$7	50

1879			1880		
Jan 25 To Balance due to date	$2	50	Sept 1 By well Roller	$1	00
" Pres & med Self		50	" 20 " 9 bu of Corn @ 50¢		
1880				$5	75
Aug 24 To Pres & med "Self"	10	00			
" 30 " " " "	1	50	Carried page 82		
Sept 19 " " " "	1	50	12.50		

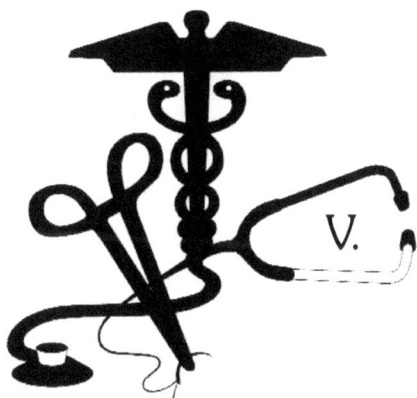

General Scoundrels

Not all of Dr. Lawrence's literary victims were condemned by him solely for ignoring his bills. There were some he just didn't like, and he often left no record as to why. Their characters must be accepted (or rejected) on faith.

In the case of some of history's greatest villains our only evidence is what one or more of their contemporaries said against them. In many cases, their enemies weren't even contemporaries. Niccolo Machiavelli is despised by people who have never read his book, or accounts of his time, but only Shakespeare's prejudices. (The same might be argued for Richard III.) Even in the case of the great Cicero, most Roman writers of his time considered him an amoral shyster—especially those in the pay of his archrival, Julius Caesar. Joan of Arc was considered a prostitute and traitor by Shakespeare and most Englishmen, until she was rehabilitated and later canonized.

Therefore, descendants of Dr. Lawrence's patients should take his comments as merely one—feisty—opinion.

For example, the 1880 note about "Newton Payne old man Slanteys brother in law," as shown on next page:

> If all the trifleing Scalawags was to wink out,
> I would guess that Newton would make his
> departure among the first
> WJC Lawrence

61

108

Charlie W. Cash.

1879   1879

1879			1879		
Apr. 1	To amount of note dated December 26th 1878, due Jan. 1st 1880, for $50.00 payable to D. M. Dean, or bearer, I traded for this today	$50.00	May 1	By Balance on Book,	
			" 25	" Balance on horse	27 50
			" 28	" Credit on harness, Dean,	5
					$40

1879   1879

| June 1 | Do Amt of Balance | $3 50 | July 4 | By W. J. B. Beall, | $35 |

1879   1879   1879

| August 12 | To Visit & medicine "Willie" | $5 00 | Dec. 21 | Charlie Cash died today and I ... that pays his account. W. J. C. Lawrence |

1879   *Newton Payne*   (Old Man Stanley's Brother)

June 5	To Call Visit & med Baby	$4 50		If all the trifling
" 6	" Visit & medicines "	4 50		Scalawags was
" 8	" " " " "	4 50		to wink out
" 11	" " " " "	4 50		I would
" 12	" " " " "	4 50		guess
	1880	$22 50		that Newton
Jan. 1	To Interest from Jan. 1st 1880			would make his departure among the first. W. J. C. Lawrence.

Similarly with one "Thomburg (at Parkins and Oquinns mill)," shown on next page:

> Old Thomburg done what all such generally does, loafed arround [sic] every where he could get and never worked so as to be of any benefit to himself or others and finally died and send his old wife back here to sponge for her living he was so awful filthy it is a wonder he did not die long before he did. [B]ut better late than never.

The word Little is surrounded with a chain of dots in one entry (page 65), entitled Little "Bob" Lee.

> If Little Robbie does not bestir himself he will more than likely deserve even a different and more closely fitting appellation than merely diminutive which now applies to principals [sic] as well as Statute [sic].

Dr. Lawrence similarly did not approve of Joseph Farras of Henderson County ($18.18), as revealed on page 66:

> Will Joeseaphus Orange Blossum is such a small fry even in his own estimation that I dislike to comment upon his qualities, they are so small, so few and so very far between that you would have to search Henderson Co over to find any established qualities he ever possessed unless it be good natured trifeling [sic] indolence.
>
> Sept 5. 1881 WJC Lawrence

Dr. Lawrence, as a product of his own time, dealt in stereotypes. There is no indication that he treated or charged those of other races differently than he did those of his own; in fact, there is internal evidence in his ledger that he treated and charged all equally. From the census of 1880, we can conclude that a large percentage of Anderson County, and therefore of his patients, were racial or ethnic minorities. At least four families in the ledger have Spanish surnames, and though African Americans are difficult to identify in the ledger, Lawrence did so three times: "Noah Bryant (Negro school teacher)," "Negro woman" at W. M. Hardyman's, and Easter and Nat Miller.

No derogatory comments were made in any of the entries. Lawrence's testimentary on the last family might seem condescending today, but was kind and trusting, compared to his opinions of other patients.

105

1879   Thornburg   (at Carturo & Equinno Mill)

Jan. 13   To Visit & medicine   Self $4 50

Old Thornburg done what all such generally does, loafed around every place he could get and never worked so as to be of any benefit to himself or others and finally died and send his old wife back here to sponge for her living he was doing filthy, it is a wonder he did not die long before he did, but better late than never.

        J. C. Lawrence

1879   Gose, Lavassa.

Feb. 6   To Visit & med   Lady $3 00   1879
               $3 00   Nov 10   By Cash $3 00
                                             $3 00

1880   1880   1880

Jan. 1   To Visit & Med.   "Baby" $3 00   Dec. 10   By Cash $18 00
"   1   " Visit & med. "Night"   "   3 00
"   2   "   "   "   "   3 00
"   3   "   "   "   "   3 00
"   8   "   "   " Men   Self   3 00
"   24   "   "   " Med.   "   3 00
                       $18 00 $18 00

1881
Apr. 5   To Pow & med.   "Ralph" $1 00
"   10   " Visit "   "   "Self"   5 00
"   12   " Done medicines   "   1 00
"   14   " Visit & meds   "   5 00

133

1880. James. Herrington. *1881*

1880					1881			
June,	17	To Visit & med. "Lady"	$3	50	Feb. 4	By Cash.	$21	00
"	25	" Pres. & med. "	1	50				
		" Visit & med. Self	3	50		Some people do not like him and insist		
		" Pres. & med. "	1	50		upon saying hard things about him but I have always found him		
		" Amt of J. A. Lawrence a/c	11	00		punctual, reliable, & kind every man has his faults and I know few		
			$21	00		worse ones than himself in my opinion. H H L $21		00

"Little" "Bob." "Lee."

1880

							If little Robbie does not better himself
June	2	To Pres. & med. "Self"	$5	00			he will more than likely deserve even
"	3	" Visit better night ?	5	00			a different and more closely fitting appel-
"	4	" " & med. "	5	00			lation than merely diminutive which now
"	6	" " " " "	5	00			applies to principals as well as Statute.
			$20	00			H. E. Lawrence
		To Interest from Jan 1 1881					
		1881					
Feb.	25	To Amt of Note 10 ⅞	$20	00			
		" Interest — at 10 %	2	00			
Apr.	13	" Pres. & med. "Lady"	1	50			

185

James, J. Wilborne

1877   1877

1877						
June 17	To Visit & Medicine arm & son	$5	00	Nov 2	By Cash	$7 50
" 18	" " to son	2	50			
Sept						
		$7	50			$7 50

Joseph L. Farrar

1877   1877

1877					1877		
June 18	To Visit & Med. Wife	$3	50	Dec 1	By 308 lb Cotton 2 25	$18	18
July 24	" " " Four Children	6	50				
Sept 12	Vis & Med Son Belfitt	1	00		Rendered at $20 00		
" 21	" " " Wife	1	00				
Oct 2	" " " Child	1	50				
" 31	Visit " Son	7	00				
"	" " " "	7	00				
"	" " " "	7					
	$8 8						
Oct 16	Visit & Med Lady	8	00				
1879							
	Visit & Med Child	1					

Sept 5, 1881   W. J. G. Laurence

Old Nat Miller stands for this acc. and agrees to pay it as soon as he gathers his crop this fall (1879).

Old Easter has gone where the good Darkies go.

This last sentence is a quote from Stephen Foster's popular song "Uncle Ned" and does not reflect yet another category within the afterlife like those Lawrence often made up as he went along. There is no indication if the Miller bill was ever paid.

Nevertheless, the common stereotype of blacks was pervasive and mean, as shown in the conclusion of Dr. Lawrence's entry condemning (the white male) France Moon, on next page:

> I have seen men of all sizes, shapes, colors, constitutions, principals [sic], temper[aments,] idiosycrases [sic] and occupations, but now I have found the appex [sic] climax a period, here is one, as utterly [sic] and entirely devoid of *any* as there are negroes who will not Steal a chicken or a fat pig.
>
> Sept 1st. 1879 WJC Lawrence.

Despite Lawrence's general conformity in racial views, he formed his own judgments of his individual patients, often at variance with the public, as he did in his entry on James Herrington (1881):

> Some people do not like Jim and insist upon saying hard things about him but I have always found him punctual, reliable, and kind. [E]very man has his faults and some have worse ones than Jim in my opinion. W.J.C.L.

Perhaps Lawrence followed the eighteenth-century example of Jonathan Swift, loathing "mankind" (and all subgroups thereof), but liking "The occasional Tom, Dick, or Harry."

In support of that supposition, the longest and most detailed account in Dr. Lawrence's ledger concerning his diagnosis, his treatments, and his patients' character is in the entry on Frank Cantrell (1881).

During his moving narrative (see page 70) Lawrence expounded on his admiration for Cantrell and his wife and sorrow for their palpable suffering, though he could not resist a side-swipe at the "skeaming [sic], swindling rascals" who were taking advantage of Cantrell's honesty. Clearly, Lawrence had found a family to revere as much as his own:

> *Frank has paid me and I have paid him all to date.* Know all that Frank Cantrell is an exception amoung [sic] all the young men arround [sic] here and that if he always adheres to the principals [sic] he now has he will live to be respected and although poor will go down to his grave respected and regretted, and he is blessed with a true, loving, virtuous and indeed a little lady for a wife. and had I not stuck to her case (post partum hemorrhage) as I did and she held up with the fortitude she

192

Pence, Moore,

I have seen men of all sizes, shapes, colors, constitutions, principals, temperaments, idiosyncrasies and occupations, but now I have found the apex, climax & period. Here is one, as utterly and entirely devoid of any — Is there one negroes who will not steal a chicken or a fat-pig.

Sept. 1st 1879.

139

1880   Frank. Cantrell.   *1881*

Oct.	13	To Pre & Med. Self	$3	60
Nov.	19	" attention and account, Lady	20	00
"	23	" Pres & Med	3	00
"	24	" " "	3	00
"	26	" " "	3	00
"	27	" " "	3	00
Dec.	7	" " "	4	00
"	12	" " "	3	00
"	13	" " "	3	00
"	14	" " "	3	00
"	15	" " "	3	00
			53	50
1881				
Jan.	1	To Interest from Jan 1881		
June	12	" Amount T.L. Wallace jr.	15	00
"	12	" Cash	1	00
Nov.	24	" "	5	50
			75	00

June	12	By One Mare	$75.00

Know all that Frank Cantrell is a ... respect..
among all the young men around here and th..t..if
he always adheres to the principals he now has
he will live to be respected and although poor
will go down to his grave respected & regretted,
and he is blessed with a true, loving, virtuous, &
indeed a little lady for a wife.. and had I not Much
to his own (Post partum hemorrhage) as I did and the
half of what the fortitude she evinced, she would certainly
have crossed the river for everything went to increase her danger
the uterus was attended with hemorrhage, requiring the introduction of my entire hand to detatch the placenta which
she bore with as much fortitude as I ever early and
... not... even during the severe operation or at any time while
she was laboring under a severe attack of Puerperal Peritonitis did she ever murmur or complain not with-
standing she was in a little log hut, cracks all open, floor open and very loose, which caused the bed to shake every time
a person crossed the room, weather extremely cold, snow on the ground all the time, She was resigned and
took everything for the best, and Poor Frank was having chills all the time and as weak he could scarcely go at all
yet he cut and packed upon his shoulders all the wood he could get into that large fire place and kept a rousing
fire night and day and set up and attended to his wifes wants giving medicines ×c, or nodded in a
chair beside her bed from the 19th of November until the 10th of January following 1881 nearly two months
and the commendable part, paid his Dr. bill as soon as he could by giving me his mare & paying the difference
and also allowed an account for medical attendance to his wife rendered three or four years previous to (come)
on, because he thought Poor Wallace Ella's father would not pay, as he had not. If I was ever to
see Frank or his family in trouble or needing money or any thing else to e...l..t him
I would never fear letting him have any thing I had for he would pay me as
soon as he promised or sooner, for Frank is an honorably high toned, honest
gentleman, and one to who has been badly treated and swindled, and being
young was persuaded by scheming spindling rascals to make trades
and that against the advice of his older brothers, which trades
turned out as every man disinterested knew they would, by the
other parties getting all and poor Frank turned out without any thing
but it never done one of them any good at least to take the poor boys home and all
as he had done several others I could mention. W. D. Lawrence

Frank has paid me & I have paid him all to date.

evinced, She would certainly have crossed the river for everything went to increase her danger the retention was attended with hemorrhage, requiring the introduction of my entire hand to detach the placenta which she bore with as much fortitude as I ever saw; and not even during the severe operation or at any time while she was laboring under a severe attack of "Puerpual [sic] Peritonitis" did she ever murmur or complain, notwithstanding she was in a little log hut, cracks all open, floor open and very loose, which caused the bed to shake every time a person crossed the room weather extremely cold. Snow on the ground all the time. She was resigned and took everything for the best, and poor Frank was having chills all the time and so weak he could scarcely go at all yet he cut and packed upon his shoulders all the wood he could get into that large fiar [sic] place and kept a rousing fiar [sic] night and day and sit up and attended to his wifes wants giving medicines and, or nodded in a chair beside her bed from the 19th of November until the 10th of January following 1881, nearly two months. and the commendable part, paid his Dr. bill as soon as he could by giving me his mare paying the difference and also allowed an account for medical attendance to his wife rendered three or four years previous to come in, because he thought Tom Wallace Ella's father would not pay it, as he had not. If I was ever to see Frank or his family in trouble or needing money or anything else to assist him I would never fear letting him have anything I had for he would pay me as soon as he promised or sooner. for Frank is an honorable, higtoned [sic], honest gentleman. And one to who has been badly treated, and swindled, and being young was persuaded by skeaming [sic] swindling rascals to make trades and that *against the advice of his older brothers,* which trades turned out as every *man* disinterested knew they would by the other parties getting all and poor Frank turned out without anything. But it never done one of them any good at least to take the poor boys home and all as he had done several others I could mention. W. J. C. Lawrence

All this about a three-by-four-inch account for "attention" and "visits" to "Lady." Clearly, Dr. Lawrence had a capacity for empathy as great as his more frequently expressed contempt.

VI.

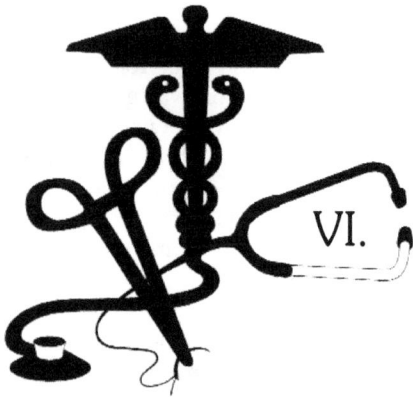

Trousers
and Death

The elderly have often believed in a Golden Age in the past, when things were better: Men were men, women were women, honor and virtue were in vogue, and prices were reasonable. This preference for the past is a venerable faith; it was shared by Cicero, Shakespeare, Spengler, and countless others. It has been argued (most recently by A. N. Wilson) that this pessimism toward the future and veneration for the past was not merely nostalgia, but based on the Christian belief in the "degeneration of generations": That each historical era takes the human community farther from the moment of Revelation, so that "in wisdom, father always trumps son." Southerners are particularly susceptible to this philosophy, living in the "Bible Belt" and being the only Americans to have ever been conquered in war, and had their way of life, right or wrong, abruptly destroyed.

A contrary belief developed in Europe among modern historians and philosophers, beginning with Gibbon, Hume, and Kant, who debunked Christianity. This led to Hegel's notion of continual progress through the "historical imperative" or "dialectic," on which Karl Marx later chose to base his theory of "dialectical materialism." On the whole, of course, Americans didn't read these modern (and modernist) European philosophers. But like all ideas, they drifted over the water and down to the people; in the case of Americans, through Ralph Waldo

Emerson, Walt Whitman, Mark Twain, the popularizations of Darwin and Freud, and through the schoolteachers who read them and passed their opinions on almost unconsciously.

The idea of perpetual progress often found fertile soil in America before the War Between the States—and in the North, since—where modern improvements were everywhere in evidence, and the community thought of itself as perpetually young and growing. Many Americans shared the faith that "progress"—whether technological inventions, universal education, economic improvement, political changes, or some other form of evolution—would lead us to the perfection of mankind and human civilization. And teachers drilled their students with repeated recitations that every day, in every way, things were getting better and better.

Adherents to the latter world-view are increasing among popular and revisionist historians. Progressivism can be a form of pride which breeds contempt for those who went before. The hardest obstacle for the most sincere historians is to put themselves in the shoes (and minds) of people in other times. It should not be surprising that we now have the paradox of historians who despise their own chosen field: the past and its people. Their condemnations include examples as varied as the Spanish Inquisition, sectarian wars, racial injustice—even the stench of horse-droppings on city streets in the nineteenth century. The wholesale horrors of the twentieth century haven't dampened the ardor of their progressivism. As G. K. Chesterton asked of the modern world, how does one know if one is living in the "Dark Ages"?

Whole careers are now built on creating and continuing the debate over the sins of our fathers, and orphaning the American people.

There is a reason that Sir Walter Scott, glorifier of the past, and Edgar Allan Poe, chronicler of loss, decay, and destruction, were the most popular poets in the South, at roughly the same time that Walt Whitman, the cheerleader for the "New Man," was the most popular poet in the triumphant North.

Unbiased historians follow one theory about the condition of virtue among people of a past time and place: That consistent (if sometimes hypocritical) denunciation of specific sins by the contemporaries of the offenders indicates a general consensus on morality—it implies that a particular civilization is made up of people who consider such evils intolerable, and exceptions to the rule.

Maybe the oldsters were right, and there was, if not exactly a Golden Age, at least one with the remnants of some virtues from which we could learn.

For all of his cynicism, Dr. William Joseph Calhoun Lawrence reflected his times. He denounced many of his own patients; however, we can conclude that their alleged offenses were exceptions, or he would not have bothered to record them.

All of his criticisms detailed above were written in a 222-page ledger, almost every page of which recorded the accounts of at least two (and often three) different patients and their families. His negative comments were the only ones about the more than 500 families he recorded, leaving the implication that the vast majority of Dr. Lawrence's patients were held in esteem by the good doctor, whose respect was not easily earned.

We can also deduce which human failings were believed to be most despicable in his day and region: failure to pay one's debts, mistreatment of one's "women-folk," cowardice (physicial or moral), theft, sloth, sexual promiscuity, lying, cheating, stinginess, prodigality, failure to teach virtue to one's children—in short, not taking responsibility for one's own actions, one's family, or for the upbringing of one's offspring. If these failings were considered exceptionable at the time of Dr. Lawrence's ledger, then we must conclude that, at least in Anderson County, their absence was the rule.

Standing on one's honor, on the other hand, was not considered a sin in 1880s Texas, and it brought an end to Dr. William Joseph Calhoun Lawrence.

Despite maintaining a medical office and a general store in Palestine, he continued his circuit-riding around the county and parts of Henderson County as well. Returning from his visits, he often passed through the village of Neches, where a Mr. L. V. Simpson, Lawrence's "cousin," owned a dry-goods store.

W. J. C. Lawrence's uncle, Dr. Josiah Allison Lawrence, had a daughter, Mary H. Lawrence, who married Mr. Simpson. The latter was therefore Calhoun Lawrence's first cousin by marriage, though Simpson's wife had died in 1881. It was therefore natural for Dr. Lawrence to pick up items at his kinsman's store during his circuits, and to maintain an account there.

For several months in the autumn of 1884, Dr. Lawrence began to notice the entry of a pair of boys' trousers in his monthly bill from that store. He remonstrated that he had never purchased such—he did not even have a son or servant who could have worn them. The arguments between Lawrence and Simpson escalated, and neither seemed willing to back down. They must have kept this quarrel somewhat private, since the *Galveston Daily News*, which reported the outcome in two editions afterwards, recorded that they were unknown to have any enmity between them.

On the morning of December 2, 1884, Dr. Lawrence announced to his wife and daughter that he was going to Neches to pay the alleged debt ($1), but, one can imagine, with bitter exclamations against his treacherous kinsman. After writing in his ledger for years about the iniquity of not paying one's bills, it would have been out of character for Lawrence to have allowed even a single person to believe or claim that Lawrence himself was guilty of such a sin. His pride, noted by all who knew him, would not have permitted.

On that day he undoubtedly wore the woolen vested suit common to all gentlemen of the time, with a double-action, .38-caliber Colt "Lightning" revolver in his pocket. This last was unremarkable: almost all men traveled armed, though not with the showy gunbelts and quick-draw holsters popularized in movie legend. This was, after all, East Texas, which was no longer the rowdy frontier. But it would have been foolhardy for a frequent traveler like Lawrence to be unarmed.

Accounts of some of the details differ, but the witnesses agreed on the essential facts when interviewed by the correspondent for the *Galveston Daily News*.

Dr. Lawrence entered Simpson's dry-goods store about 4:15 P.M., while other customers were there. Whatever Lawrence's original purpose, he and Simpson resumed their argument, and Lawrence made the fatal, if inevitable, error of charging Simpson with cowardice. Simpson then brought out a revolver. Someone shouted, "Look out, Doc!" and Simpson told Lawrence to defend himself. Lawrence immediately drew his own revolver.

The *Galveston Daily News* account of December 3 ("START-
LING DOUBLE TRAGEDY AT NECHES") says that Simpson fired the
first shot. The witnesses, responding to questions from both
families, agreed, and this is the most likely version, though perhaps irrelevant considering all the circumstances. Nevertheless,
the follow-up *News* account given on the 4th ("FURTHER PARTIC-
ULARS OF THE NECHESVILLE DOUBLE KILLING") contradicts its
original version, and describes the shootout in a style reminiscent of the dime novels of the period, though it is presumably
more accurate:

> Lawrence fired the first shot, which took effect near Simpson's
> heart. The latter then fired, striking Lawrence in the breast.
> They then emptied their pistols at each other, nearly every
> shot taking effect. When Simpson had emptied his pistol he
> struck Lawrence over the head with it and turned and fell
> dead. Simpson's first wound was almost instantly fatal, and
> that he lived to fire his remaining shots is wonderful.

For Simpson to have hit Lawrence with the barrel or the
butt, considering the short length of the pistols, the antagonists
must have been face-to-face.

According to the *News*, Lawrence, despite all the bullet holes
and the pistol-whipping, then walked into a nearby store before
falling down. He was taken to his brother-in-law's house, where
he lived until 6:00 P.M. Dying, he "begged that Simpson's body
should be brought by his side, and when it was done he be-
moaned his rash act, saying he was sorry he had killed poor
Simpson." The *News* called Lawrence "a young man of good family" and "a rising physician," and added that, "Both had many
friends and the sad and tragic affair is generally deplored."

It cannot be denied that both men had remarkably strong
constitutions.

An ironical twist, which Dr. Lawrence might have appreci-
ated, was that the two revolvers involved were a matched set,
given separately to each of the cousins.

Many years later a mystery surfaced as to whether the "boys'
trousers" were the real cause of the feud and bloody shootout.
The principals were in no condition to shed light on the mystery, and neither family ever said or wrote anything about it
afterwards. But a letter has emerged which strongly implies that,

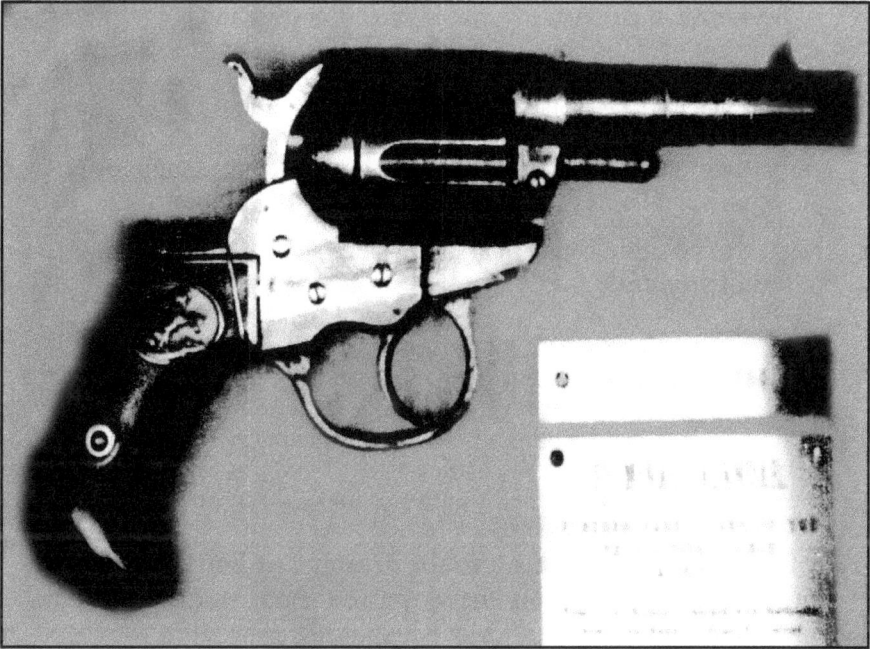

A revolver with an ironical twist.
— Courtesy of Egon Richard Tausch

the *Galveston News* to the contrary, a hatred arose between the men a year and a half before the shootout, and a year before the "trousers" bill arrived.

Dr. Lawrence wrote to his wife, on the stationery of his dry-goods store, a letter dated June 26, 1883. It stated that he was writing from the village of Neches, where Simpson lived and worked, and first described threads, needles, merchants he visited, etc. He consoled Fannie and "Little Baby May," repeatedly, for his absence and their loneliness. He then indicated, apparently for the first time, his interest in moving to another part of the country, even at great financial loss:

> . . . .As soon as we get a little better off I intend taking you where you can be more in Company and with nice people, but we must endure it for a year or two longer unless we can sell out our lands which would enable us to go sooner but if we can not sell I think that in a couple of years more if we have no bad

luck we can go any way even if we can not sell the lands, and have enough to begin business as well as to buy us a nice home. Then we will be glad won't we May? Mama will be too when she get to a new place, and has nice new home Conveniant [sic] to Good Schools, Churches, Neighbors, and Good Society, at least she will be after she is there long enough to be acquainted. Won't you dear? I think you will!

Then the possible cause of such anxiety to relocate comes up, as an "afterthought":

> . . . .One thing would like to ask you, to treat *Simpson, Cooly* [sic] *polite,* but not to have any more to say to him than etiquet [sic] demands, at a friends house, but under no circumstances be seen out in his company, or even appear very friendly with him . . . will tell you my reason when I see you and they are good ones, or of course I would not make this request.

If Lawrence ever told his wife the reason that her family should shun Cousin Simpson, she never passed it on. Nor did Dr. Lawrence live long enough to move his family away from the vicinity. The obloquy implied by Dr. Lawrence's letter cannot have been caused by any of the usual vices which devout Methodist gentlemen might have ascribed to others—Lawrence's best customers were heavy drinkers, and there was no dearth of womanizers, deadbeats, or even thieves among his patients and acquaintances. It probably lies in his obsessive concern for his wife and family, and in his own overblown sense of personal honor.

The entire mystery seems to reflect the unwritten laws of the duel: The actual cause is never revealed (it could besmirch a lady's reputation), but instead a false quarrel is invented; traditionally a glove slapped across a face. Thus, most duels left mysteries forever unsolved. It appears that even this untidy Texas shootout follows the pattern, though an invoice for boys' trousers doesn't seem to have the panache of a thrown gauntlet or glove-slap.

If this speculation is correct, it still does not imply that both Simpson and Lawrence knew the real cause of the killings: Either man could have intentionally provoked the other, through repeated needling about the $1.00 invoice or anything else, knowing that his antagonist could eventually be driven to violence, for which he himself would be prepared. Or think he was prepared.

Death, however mourned at the time, was not the universally feared and loathed phenomenon it seems to have become in later years. There was no resulting family feud or bitterness; the extended families of both men grieved together, and remained on (or reverted to) good terms.

Even the lawyers stayed out of it.

Fannie Mae Lawrence mourned her loss, gave birth to Dr. Lawrence's daughter, whom she named after him, and in May of 1887 she married Dr. Frank B. Moore, who had been best man at Calhoun's wedding to Fannie Mae, and who had assumed most of Lawrence's medical practice after his death.

Dr. William Joseph Calhoun Lawrence would have been happy that his "Darling and Little Ducklings" were well cared for.

Some things were not so quickly or easily forgiven and forgotten, especially within a family as steeped in the Southern experience as the families and friends of Calhoun and Fannie Mae. Dr. Lawrence's daughter, Leta Clementine, chose to marry James Harvey Briggs III, the son of an oilman.

Though he grew up in Texas, Briggs happened to be of Northern (specifically, Puritan New England) extraction. His nickname at West Texas Military Academy (now Texas Military Institute) in San Antonio was "Bluebelly." Thus all Dr. Lawrence's descendants would have at least some Northern blood. In disgust, the now twice-widowed Fannie Mae Lawrence Moore boycotted her daughter's wedding.

Despite the absence of male children, and the infusion of "tainted blood," the Lawrence family names did not completely die out. Dr. Lawrence's granddaughter, Frances Lawrence Briggs (Tausch) carried on both Calhoun's and Fannie Mae's names; *her* daughter, Frances Clementine, was named after both Fannie Mae and the numerous "Clementines" in the clan, while her son, the editor of this ledger, named his only child Mary Lawrence.

May individuality, eccentricity, and strong character never disappear among those peculiar people called Texans.

Appendix

Patients Recorded in
Dr. Lawrence's Ledger
(Spelling according to Dr. Lawrence)

Adams, Gus
Addington, M. H.
Allen, Curry
  (at the Merrytt place)
Allen, Mr. & Mrs. N. G.
  (at the Merrytt place)
Allen, Oscar
Allen, W.P.
Allen, William
Allen, Willie
  (at the Merrytt place)
Atwood, Mr. & Mrs. "Bud"
Atwood, Felix
Atwood, Louis
Bagwell, Aenic
  (at John Hallum's)
Bagwell, Henry
  (at John Hallum's)
Bailey, Mr. & Mrs. Fred
  (at Griffin Hamilton's)
Bailey, Johnson
  (at Griffin Hamilton's)
Bailey, Sallie
  (at Griffin Hamilton's)
Banks, Mr. & Mrs. Linsey
  (at Maudica Hardman's)
Barber, Bill
Beall, Addie
Beall, Harriet
Beall, Hattie
Beall, Mr. & Mrs. W. J. S.
Beall, Whiten
Beall, Willie

Benson, John H.
Bizell, Mrs.
  (at Dr. Miller's place)
Blansit, Mr. & Mrs. Calvin
Blansit, Joe
Blount, Rev. & Mrs. B. F.
Blount, B. F. Jr.
Blount, Bula
Blount, Eddie
Blount, Edna
Blount, Mr. & Mrs. Eugenius
Blount, Imogene
Bobbitt, Mr. & Mrs. Bill
Bone, Nattie
Bone, S. V.
Boosier, Nelson
Booth, Dora
Booth, Henry
Booth, Hubbard
Booth, Rev. Thomas Trussvan
Bradford, George
  (at I.R. Emerson's)
Brooks, Jim
  (at John Cely's)
Brooks, Mariah
  (at John Cely's)
Brooster, James M.
Brown, Dave
Brown, Mrs.
  (Mother of Dave Brown)
Brown, Dick
Brown, Eliza Willi
Brown, Mr. & Mrs. John W.

Brown, Mr. & Mrs. John W.
Brown, Mariah
Brown, Sharlott
Brown, Young
Bryant, Bob
Bryant, Noah O.
Burgamy, Mr. & Mrs. Emery
Burgamy, Mr. & Mrs. Mat
Busby, Mr. & Mrs. Anderson
Busby, Hode
    (at W.R. Clanahan's)
Caldwell, James S.
Caldwell, Lula
Caldwell, Robert
Caldwell, Sallie
Calhoun, R.W.
Cantrell, Annie
Cantrell, Effie
Cantrell, Mr. & Mrs. Frank
Cantrell, John
Cantrell, Mr. & Mrs. S.J. "Dock"
Cantrell, Mr. & Mrs. Shade
Cantrell, Stella
Cantrell, Susie
Cappes, Mr. & Mrs. Anderson M.
Cappes, Jack
Carroll, Abna M.
Carroll, Henry
Carroll, Woodley
Cary, Sydna
Cash, Charlie W.
Cash, Willis
Cely, Billy
Cely, Mr. & Mrs. John T.
Cely, Sady
Clanahan, "Uncle" Jimmie
Clanahan, Mr. & Mrs. William
Chamblee, Mit
    (at Old Lady Taylor's)
Chamblee, Tom
    (at Old Lady Taylor's)
Coleman, Jim
Coleman, Mary Ann
Colley, Mr. & Mrs. John
Colley, Thomas
Colley, Mrs.
    (Mother of Thomas Colley)
Colley, Willie

Colvin, Alabam
    (at Parson Blount's)
Colvin, Mr. & Mrs. Peter
    (at Parson Blount's)
Condus, Mr. & Mrs. Poince
Cook, A. Young
Corder, Mrs. A. C.
Corder, Mr. & Mrs. Curtis
Corder, Lavinia
Costeloe, George
Cowden, Willie
Cunningham, James
Curtis, Mr. & Mrs. Henry
Daves, Jim
Dean, Bulah
Dean, Mr. & Mrs. Harrison
Dennis, Sallie
Devers, Sophrona
    (Mrs. Doughty's niece)
Dickerson, Rheubin
Donnell, Daniel
Donnell, Phillip
    (Allen Johnson's brother-in-law)
Donnell, Tobe
    (at Gus Dickson's)
Doss, Joe
Doss, S. P.
    (at Addington's)
Doughty, Earl
Doughty, Edna
Doughty, Ferdinand F.
Doughty, Mr. & Mrs. Henry P.
Doughty, Mr. & Mrs. Henry T.
Dowell, Mr. & Mrs. K.
    (at Slammies)
Dunlap, Nathan G.
Duvall, Killis
Duvall, Mr. & Mrs. Neil
    (Garland Reynold's grandson)
Duvall, Matton
Elkins, Barton
Elkins, Johnnie
Elkins, Rev. & Mrs. M. G.
Elkins, William
Emerson, Charley
Emerson, Green
Emerson, Harland
Emerson, I. Read

Emerson, "Little" Read
Emerson, Mr. & Mrs. J. Read
Emerson, James M.
Emerson, May
Emerson, Nona
Emerson, Oren
Emerson, Sallie
England, E.
  (at Sharp place)
Evens, Billy
Evens, Dave
Evens, "Little" Dave
Evens, Dosie
Evens, Ella
Evens, Mr. & Mrs. Jim
Evens, Josie
Evens, Ludie
  (nee Beachamp)
Evens, Lusk
Evens, Mimmie
Evens, Mr. & Mrs. Sam
Fair, Beck
Fair, Mr. & Mrs. Charles
Falk, Mr. & Mrs. Henry
Fane, Mr. & Mrs. Bob
Farras, Mr. & Mrs. Joseph
Farras, Tom
Featherstone, James
Foscue, Mr. & Mrs. Billy
Foster, Demsa
Foster, Johnie
Fowler, Rev. & Mrs. Littleton M.
Freeman, George
  (old man Frank Oldham's grand-
  son)
Furlon, Mr. & Mrs. Dallas
Gaddis, Charlie
  (at William Herrington Jr.'s)
Gaines, Mit
Gaines, Noble
Gaines, Mr. & Mrs. Thomas
Galaway, Dick
  (at John Cely's)
Galaway, Emma
  (at John Cely's)
Galaway, Mr. & Mrs. W. Harrison
  (at John Cely's)
Gentry, Mr. & Mrs. James

  (at Tom Mope's)
Givens, Katie
Givens, William
Givens, Sam
Gore, William
Graham, Granbery
Graham, Mr. & Mrs. R. C.
  (at Parker's & Oquinn's Mill)
Green, Rev. Henry Sr.
Green, Mr. & Mrs. Jerry
  (at J. M. Emerson's)
Green, Willis
Gregg, A. White
Gregg, Bennet
Griffin, Charlie
Griffin, Mr. W.L.
  (Mrs. Goley's "old man")
Griffin, Winnie
Grinnin, Lucy
Hallum, Anderson
Hallum, John
Hallum, (Negro) John
Hallum, Morris
  (at James Y. Wilborn's)
Hallum, nona
Hallum, Stewart
Hamilton, Ann
Hamilton, Mr. & Mrs. Elias
Hamilton, George
Hamilton, I. Griffin
Hamilton, John
Hamilton, Mary
Hamilton, Mr. & Mrs. Perry
Hamilton, Mr. & Mrs. W. Ira
Hancock, Mr. & Mrs. G. A.
Hardman, Arthur
Hardman, Mr. & Mrs. Blueford
Hardman, Calhoun
Hardman, Dennis
Hardman, Frank
Hardman, Homer
Hardman, Newton
Hardman, Maudica
Hardman, Warna
Hardman, "Little" Warna
Hardman, Willi
Harris, Mr. & Mrs. Charley
Harris, Lina

(Charley Harris' sister)
Harten, Mr. & Mrs. Walker L.
Hawk, Charlie
Hawk, Mr. & Mrs. J.
Hayes, James E.
Henderson, Mr. & Mrs. Ben
Henderson, Mr. & Mrs. Daniel
Henderson, Don
Henderson, Dora
Henderson, Harrison
Henderson, Mr. & Mrs. Henry
Henderson, Leah
Henderson, Lona
Henderson, Mollie
Henry, Mrs. A. J.
Henry, Mr. & Mrs. Issac
Henry, "Little" Ike
Herrington, Mr. & Mrs. Allen
Herrington, Mr. & Mrs. E.
Herrington, Ella
Herrington, Henry
Herrington, Mr. & Mrs. James
Herrington, Ida
Herrington, Jim
Herrington, Laura
Herrington, Lizzie
Herrington, Rufus
Herrington, Sam
Herrington, Mr.&Mrs. William Jr.
Herrington, William Sr.
Hiner, John
Hiner, Ruth
Hinsley, J. M.
    (at John Cely's)
Hodge, Mr. & Mrs. Robert
Hollingstead, Mr. & Mrs.
    (at "old man" Thomells)
Hollis, Mr. & Mrs. James
Holt, Thomas
Hopper, Mr. & Mrs. John
Horton, Mr. & Mrs. Woodley
House, Mr. & Mrs. George
Hughes, Mr. & Mrs. Louis
Hyett, Mr. & Mrs. W.R.
Jasper, Mr. & Mrs. George
Jefferson, Solomon
Jeeter, Mr. & Mrs. Buck
Johnson, Alice

Johnson, Allen
Johnson, Ben
Johnson, Betty
Johnson, Clarra
Johnson, Jack
    (at A.J. Wylies)
Johnson, Jessee
Johnson, Leah
Johnson, Noble
Johnson, Phil
Johnson, Sam
    (at Mrs. Brown's place)
Jones, James
    (Duff Jones' brother)
Lane, Mr. & Mrs.
    (Givens' brother-in-law)
Lavassa, Mr. & Mrs. Bob "Bud"
Lavassa, Mr. & Mrs. Gofe
Lavassa, Ralph
Lawrence, Mary Clementine
Lee, "Big" Bob
Lee, Mr. & Mrs. "Little" Bob
Lee, George
Lee, J. Henry
Lee, Rhoulen
    (at Jim Herrington's)
Lightfoot, George
Lightfoot, Jim
Lightfoot, Willie
Loftlin, Mr. & Mrs. James
Loftlin, Sallie
Louis, Mr. & Mrs. Larkin
    (at Henry Henderson's place)
Lusk, Albert M.D.C.
Lynch, Mr. & Mrs.
Marriner, Mr. & Mrs. John
    (near "Mrs. Dr." Miller's)
Martin, Anderson
    (alias "Hallum")
Mathews, Melia
McFarline, Mr. & Mrs. Rhube C.
McGuire, Thomas
    (Capp's brother-in-law)
McInish, Allen
    (allias "Wadkins")
McInish, "Uncle" John
McMillin, Andrew
Meyers, Henry

Meyers, William
Michium, Eliza
Michium, Washington
Miller, Easter
Miller, George
  (allias "Caddo")
Miller, John A.
Miller, Mrs. L.A.
Miller, Mr. & Mrs. Nat
Miller, Mr. & Mrs. Wiley
Millin, Jim
Millin, Minnie
Millner, Charley
Millner, Maud
Millner, Mr. & Mrs. Thomas
Milner, Charles
Milner, Mr. & Mrs. George W.
Moon, France M.
Moon, Jack
Moon, Mr. & Mrs. Jessee J.
Moon, Mr. & Mrs. L. M. B.
Moore, Frank
Moore, Mr. & Mrs. James
  (at G. W. Milner's)
Moore, W. A.
Mop, Eliza
Mop, Jodie
Mop, Joe
Mop, John
Mop, "Old" John
Mop, Rattie
Mop, Stephen
Mop, Mr. & Mrs. Tone
Morfatt, Marion
  (Buck Jeeter's brother-in-law)
Morgan, Mr. & Mrs. James
Morow, Rev. Robert R.
Morrorr, Dave
  (son-in-law of Mrs. Taylor)
Morrorr, Elijah
Moss, Eliza
Moss, Mr. & Mrs. Frank
Moss, George
Moss, Harriet
Moss, Laura
Moss, Mariah
Moss, Mat
Moss, Mr. & Mrs. William F.

Murphy, Bela
Murphy, Mat
Night, Mr. & Mrs. Jack
Norwood, William W.
Oldham, Frank Sr.
Oquinn, Mr. & Mrs. Lum
Oquinn, Maudy
Oquinn, Mr. & Mrs. Rufus
Oquinn, Tenny
Overby, John
Overby, Mr. & Mrs. Pleasant
Pace, Lulla
Pace, "Old Man"
  (O. D. Pace's father)
Pagitt, Bob
Pagitt, Mr. & Mrs. Joseph
Pagitt, Mr. & Mrs. Pleasant
Pagitt, Mr. & Mrs. Robert
Palmer, Dina
Palmer, Narcis
Palmer, Welton
Parker, Rhodie
Parker, Mrs. Russell S.
Parker, Mr. & Mrs. Silas M.
Patterson, Agustus
Patterson, John W.
Paul, Sam
Payne, Newton
  (brother-in-law of Mr. Stanley)
Payne, Samuel
Peter, Calvin
  (at Mr. Blount's)
Pickle, Mr. & Mrs. Charley
Porter, "Widow"
Prewitt, Eddie
Prewitt, Mr. & Mrs. James
Prewitt, Willie
Reynolds, Dosia
  (Ned Reynolds' wife)
Reynolds, Garland
Reynolds, George
Reynolds, Laura
Reynolds, Mimmie
Reynolds, Nelson
Reynolds, Pleasant
Reynolds, Tempie
Rhodes, George
Rhodes, Hattie

Rhodes, Mr. & Mrs. Houston
Rhodes, Hudgens
Rhodes, John
Rhodes, Porter
Richards, Mr. & Mrs. Benny
Richards, Webster
Richardson, Mr. & Mrs. Edam
Robertson, Mr. & Mrs. Wesley
  (at Henry Henderson's)
Robinson, Mr. & Mrs. Henry
Robinson, Jenny
Robinson, Rothele
Robinson, William W.
Rodgers, Austin
Rodgers, Mr. & Mrs. Ben F.
Rodgers, Columbus
Rodgers, Scilas
Rodgers, Mr. & Mrs. Thomas
  (step-son of Columbus Rodgers &
  son-in-law of John Elrod)
Rodgers, William
  (John Daves' brother-in-law)
Ross, John
  (at Allen Johnson's)
Rushing, Bob
Rushing, Mr. & Mrs. Jack
Rushing, Sallie
Rushing, Winnie
Russel, Dickson G.
  (Parker's son-in-law)
Russey, Mr. & Mrs. Joseaphus
Russey, Willie
Saunders, Mr. & Mrs. Dave A.
Sauney, Bill
Scarborough, John Lawrence Sr.
Scarborough, Johnie
Scown, Mr. & Mrs.
  (Englishman at "Mrs. Dr."
  Miller's)
Scown, John
Scown, Tom
Sellers, J. H.
  (at Oquinn's Mill)
Semenon & Shafer
  (on my place)
Shumatt, Oren
  (at "Mrs. Dr." Miller's)
Slaughter

Slone, Clark
  (at Charles Faire's)
Slone, Ella
  (at Charles Faire's)
Slone, Nathan
  (at Charles Faire's)
Smith, J. Hillery "Dean"
  (at Addington's)
Smith, Lenora
  (at Addington's)
Smith, Newton
Smith, Mr. & Mrs. W. B.
  (Galaway's son-in-law: at "Old"
  Slammies)
Sorter, T. Cull
Soule, Frank
  (at Ben Elrod's place)
Sowell, William
Stanley, George
Stanley, Ruth
Stanley, Mr. & Mrs. William
Stephens, James S.
Stephens, Jane
Stephens, Lawrence
Stephens, Sissie
Stephens, Tonk
Stephens, Mr. & Mrs. W.K.
Stephens, Wylie
Strander, Jacob
  (at "Mrs. Doc." Miller's)
Strander, Mrs. John
  (at "Mrs. Doc." Miller's)
Swearmegin, Mr. & Mrs. John
  (at Allen Herrington's)
Tatum, Eland
Taylor, Ellen
Taylor, Frank
  (Hugh White's son-in-law)
Taylor, Mrs. P. J.
  (Mrs. Wash Taylor's)
Thomas, Annie
Thomas, Mr. & Mrs. Billy
  (Emerson's son-in-law)
Thomas, Colley
Thomas, Mrs.
  (mother of Colley Thomas)
Thomas, Green
Thomas, Johnie

Thomburg
(at Parker's & Oquinn's Mill)
Thompson, William
(William Mopes' brother-in-law)
Thornell, "Old Man"
Thornell, Charley
Thornell, Columbus C.
Thornell, Florence
Thornell, Gussie
Thornell, Ira
Thornell, Mr. & Mrs. Sidna
Thrasher
(near Parson Artists)
Tinnell, Seabin
Tippin, George
Tubbs, Granville
Tubbs, John
Tubbs, Nancy
Tubbs, Peter,
Tubbs, Sylvester
Tucker, Add
Tucker, Bill
Tucker, Frances
Tucker, Jenny
(Old George Caddoe's wife)
Tucker, Sallie
Tucker, Whit
Underhill, Jimmie
Vaugh, Mr. & Mrs. Leah
Vaughan, Joseph
(with Uncle John McInish)
Vaughan, Isiah
Wadkins, Allen
(alias McInish)
Waldroup, Mr. & Mrs. Dick
Walker, Ed
Wallace, Mary
Wallace, Mr. & Mrs. Thomas J.
Wallace, Thomas K.
Warren, Mr. & Mrs. Ab
(at Pleasant Pagitt's)
Warren, Alice
Warren, Billy
Warren, Calhoun
(at P. Pagitt's)

Warren, Mr. & Mrs. David
Warren, Mr. & Mrs. Henry
(at P. Pagitt's)
Warren, Mr. & Mrs. Will
(at P. Pagitt's)
Warren, Will
(R. B. Warren's son)
Warren, Willie
Watkins, James T.
Watkins, Jimmie
Watson, Mr. & Mrs. Allen
Watson, Henry
Watson, Kit
Watson, Ned
Watson, Rose
Webb, Allie
White, Allie
White, Mr. & Mrs. Hugh L.
White, Jerome
White, Read
White, Sudie
Willbanks, Mr. & Mrs. Abe
Wilborne, James Y.
Williams, Harrison
Williams, James
Willingham, Bell
Willingham, Johnie
Willingham, W. H.
Wood, Jacob
(Even's brother-in-law)
Woosley, Dave
Worren, "Little" Bob
Worren, Bud
Worren, John
Worren, Johnie
Worren, Parker
Worren, Mr. & Mrs. Robert B.
Worren, Tex
Wylie, Andy J.
Wylie, Etta
Wylie, G. Lee
Wylie, Tom
Young, "Capt." John

Bibliography

BOOKS

Anderson, John Q. *Texas Folk Medicine*. Austin: Encino Press, 1970.

Barker, Eugene C. *History of Texas*. Austin: University of Texas Press, 1929.

Biesele, Rudolph Leopold. *History of the German Settlements in Texas*. Austin: University of Texas, 1964.

Bower, Claude. *The Tragic Era: The Revolution After Lincoln*. Cambridge, Massachusetts: The Riverside Press, 1929.

Burnham, W. Dean. *Presidential Ballots, 1836-1892*. Baltimore: Johns Hopkins Press, 1955.

Daniel, M. D., F. E. *Recollections of a Rebel Surgeon and Other Sketches*. Austin: Von Boeckmann, Schutze & Co., 1899.

Dunlop, Richard. *Doctors of the American Frontier*. Garden City, New York: Doubleday and Company, 1962-1965.

Fehrenbach, T. R. *Lone Star*. New York: The Macmillan Company, 1968.

Ferris, Sylvia Van Voast, and Eleanor Sellers Hoppe. *Scalpels and Sabres: 19th Century Medicine in Texas*. Austin: Eakin Press, 1985.

Foote, Shelby. *The Civil War: A Narrative*. New York: Random House, 1958.

Handbook of Texas. Edited by Walter Prescott Webb, et al. Austin: Texas State Historical Association, Volumes 1 and 2, 1952; and *A Supplement*, edited by Eldon Stephen Branda, Austin: Texas State Historical Association, 1976.

Henderson, Col. Harry McCorry. *Texas in the Confederacy*. San Antonio: The Naylor Company, 1955.

Hohes, Pauline Buck. *A Centennial History of Anderson County, Texas*. San Antonio: The Naylor Press, 1936.

Hood, R. Maurice, ed. *Early Texas Physicians, 1830-1915*. Austin: State House Press, 1999.

Kingsmill, Hugh. *Anthology of Invective and Abuse*. New York: Dial Press Inc., 1929.

Masters, Edgar Lee. *Lincoln. The Man.* Originally published 1931; new edition, Columbia, South Carolina: The Foundation for American Education, 1998.

Nixon, Pat Ireland. *The Medical Story of Early Texas.* Mollie Bennett Lupe Memorial Fund, 1946.

Ramsdell, Charles William. *Reconstruction in Texas.* Gloucester, Peter Smith, 1949.

Wilson, A. N. *God's Funeral.* Horton W. W. & Co. Inc., 1999.

Winkler, William, ed. *Journal of the Secession Convention of Texas, 1861.* Austin: Austin Printing Company, 1912.

THESES, PERIODICALS, AND PAPERS

Galveston Daily News. Galveston (with various name changes), 1865-present.

Lawrence, Dr. W. J. C., medical ledger of. Unpublished.

Lawrence, Dr. W. J. C., letters of. Unpublished.

"The Peaches Portfolio." Various Lawrence descendants. Unpublished.

Trinity News (Advocate). Palestine, 1861-1875.

Tausch, Egon Richard. "Southern Sentiment Among the Texas Germans During the Civil War and Reconstruction." Master's thesis, University of Texas, Austin, 1965.

Index

www.ingramcontent.com/pod-product-compliance
Lightning Source LLC
Chambersburg PA
CBHW071607200326
41519CB00021BB/6903